Self

Ease anxi

being a ...ghly sensitive woman

By Maryse Cardin

Book cover design by Avital David

Published by Dandelion Winds Press

ISBN: 978-1-7751141-3-0

For inspiration and tools visit
www.selftalklove.com and
www.facebook.com/selftalklove

For Eloise

Highly sensitive and magnificent

Words of Praise for Self Talk Love for Sensitives

"Maryse writes with the strength to be vulnerable - this is an honest, authentic peek into what it's like to be an HSP woman, full of deep insight, inspiring stories, meaningful metaphors, and many powerfully targeted messages that empower women to replace their self doubt/ inner critic by building a loving inner voice. I think most HSPs will find this book helpful and a pleasure to savour, full of heart warming, healthy thoughts to use as tools to build self esteem. You will feel as if she's speaking personally to you, as if she deeply knows your needs. And knows what validates you."
-- **Pamela Catapia, MA, RCC. HSP Counsellor and Educator**

"Maryse manifested another great book for the Greater Good: simple and effective tools to do self-care for all highly sensitive women. Her kindness and compassion, and her beautiful journey of expansion into Oneness are accessible to all."—**Camilla Ravindran, co-author of Being Feminine: 12 invitations to anchor your gifts in daily life.**

Also by Maryse Cardin

Speaking to Yourself with Love, Transform Your Self Talk

Speaking to Yourself with Love Workbook, Transform Your Self Talk

Self Talk Love for Fertility, On Your Way to Motherhood

All Maryse's books are available at:

www.selftalklove.com and on Amazon

Introduction

Dear highly sensitive woman,

You are magnificent. There. Let's start with the truth, and the essence of who we are as highly sensitive women (HSW).

It's safe to say that if you are reading this book, you already know – or you have an inkling – that you are a highly sensitive person. You may be wondering, hey, how come I seem to feel so much more than others? How come I get overwhelmed when there are too many people, there is too much noise, or there's too much of a good thing? How come beauty, art, nature, and music touch me profoundly and break me open?

If you've often felt weird and out of sorts with the other ducklings, it's because you are a glorious HSW swan. Welcome to your real pond. Welcome to the HSW family. You have always been a member of this tribe. I say always because we are born highly sensitive – we are not made. This trait, this gift, is ours from the get-go.

This book is remarkably close to my heart because it speaks to my passion for positive and loving self talk, and it is written specifically for my favourite women of all, my highly sensitive sisters. What's there not to love?

Self Talk Love for Sensitives, Ease Anxiety and Awaken to The Gifts of Being a Highly Sensitive Woman is a collection of stories and contemplations about the nature of being an HSW. It also highlights ways that we can put our self talk in service to ourselves to soothe, to lighten, to heal, and to celebrate. Some of the stories include tips on how to transform your self talk so that your inner words become your ally. Please forgive me for this. I'm a university teacher and I can't seem to stop myself from seeing everything as a chance to grow and gain a few extra skills.

Loving self talk skills

We can use our self talk to guide ourselves towards who we want to be and what we want to create in our lives and in this world. Our inner words have so much power. Your self talk influences every cell in your body, your brain, your nervous system. It plays a role in your health, in your mood, in your outlook on life, and in your ability to manifest your dreams. It also has a big effect on whether you feel calm inside. Why not use it to your advantage?

It's like if you had a gorgeous Tesla, but you were only travelling in your old gas-guzzling, grossly polluting beater. Positive and loving self talk is your Tesla. Negative, critical, defeated, and cruel self talk is your beater. The choice is yours. The power is yours.

We can all benefit from positive and loving self talk skills. Highly sensitive people in particular benefit greatly from knowing how to do it. We feel things very deeply. We are not wired like the average person, and we need specialized care. We are not more prone to anxiety than anyone else, but if you add trauma to our sensitivity, then we become more likely to develop the condition. We are the proverbial canaries. When the environment is toxic, stressful, hard, or unkind, we feel it first and we feel it intensely.

We are sensitive by design

Highly sensitive women are not beings in need of fixer-upping. We are made like this by design. We exist in every culture and even in animals, and we always make up about the same percentage of the population. The difference is that some societies and times in history value our sensitivity more than other times and places.

The world right now is transforming, and we are needed more than ever in the creation of a new world. We are masters. Masters of care, of kindness, of healing, of intuition, of justice, of gentleness, of humour, of compassion, of wholeness, of spirituality, of power, of courage, of vision, of fairness, of beauty, of nature, and of forgiveness. We embody the qualities that the world needs to come into more balance. We are the embodiment of the new world.

What you say inside radiates out into the world. As in, as out. As your self talk transforms into love, compassion, courage, joy, and kindness, the world follows suit. A new world starts with you. You have that power. It is possible. The way you speak to yourself counts, brave one.

We are a blessing. I want us to take some moments in this book to celebrate how awesome, essential, and gifted we are. Hooray for us! Hooray for the world for having us! Hooray for those lucky enough to be in close proximity to us!

Lighten the load

Let's talk about lightening the load for a bit. As HSWs, we are able to feel what other people are feeling. Our empathy skills are in overdrive. We are the gold medal winners of empathy. We don't even have to strive for it; that muscle is just built into us. What we do need to strive for is not taking on what is not ours. We are not donkeys put upon this earth to carry other people's burdens, fears, and life lessons for them, up steep hills on treacherous muddy paths. You see where I am going here. I obviously used to think I was a mule. Let me carry this for you, I used to say. Let me take this weight for you. No problem at all. Crack! What was that? Is that my back breaking from a load I was never made to carry?

I was completely enmeshed and entangled in other people's business. Then I learned that there is such a thing as my business, and then there's your business, and finally divine's own business. I've got to focus on my own business like a captain focuses on her ship. I'm out to sea in a storm and I've got to get this ship to port. I'll give a helping hand if someone needs help, for sure. I want all the ships to come back safely. That does not mean that I abandon my ship to run someone else's. If I do that, my own ship is going to run aground. I'll be shipwrecked. And now that's enough with the sea captain analogies.

Sometimes HSPs can get lost in situations and forget that they are more important than whatever they are facing. If you'd like a reminder that you are more important than your problems, take some time with this free worksheet that you can download from my website: https://selftalklove.lpages.co/self-talk-love-i-am-more-important-than-my-problems-worksheet/

Wear and tear

Several of my vintage HSW friends developed anxiety after one too many bumps in the road, trials and tribulations like divorce, toxic relationships, single parenthood, car accidents, high-stress jobs, and financial worries. These are strong, educated, adventurous, successful, hyper-capable women. For the most part, they have soldiered through despite being anxious. They are what you'd call high-functioning.

For lack of a better way to explain it, there seems to be wear and tear that takes place. Our systems just can't seem to take what they once could without blinking an eye. I'll leave it to you to look up the science behind it. There are many excellent books on the topic.

For a while there, anxiety and I were companions. There came a point where I couldn't feel the difference between anxiety and excitement. Packing my suitcase for a trip would almost bring on a panic attack instead of a sense of enthusiasm and anticipation. My nervous system was trigger-happy. The woman who once jumped out of planes, hitchhiked in the back of pick-up trucks in Central America, and dove with sharks now got stressed throwing clothes into a suitcase.

I'm here to tell you that a nervous system can be healed. Health can be restored. Inner calm can be fostered, and you can free yourself from negative self talk.

There's so much that happens in a life, so much that is out of our control. Self talk is not one of those things. When I fall off the wagon and fall back into negative self talk, I get right back on as soon as I can. I'll tell you why. I want to be on board because I've set my wagon in the direction of self-love, self-empowerment, inner peace, and well-being.

That's my intention, that's my destination. That's who I want to be with myself and others, and that's what I want to offer the world. I don't know how long it will take to get there, but it's ok cause I'm on my way.

You, too, have the power to set your destination. Who do you want to be? How do you want to live? Your self talk can be your superpower in getting you there.

So, to recap, being highly sensitive is a trait we are born with. It comes with many gifts and some challenges that we can learn to navigate. We are not like others – just like a beautiful, fair-skinned redhead with freckles needs special care in the sun, while a Mediterranean dark beauty with olive skin may not. No one is superior to the other. We are simply different splendors. I do find us very beautiful, and if you don't feel that way now, you'll feel it by the end of this book.

I am excited for you, dear HSW. Together, let's start imagining what it would mean to speak to yourself with love, with compassion, with support; what it would be like to celebrate your exceptionality; what it would be like to put down the load that isn't yours to carry; what it would be like to bestow upon yourself the precious care you need and are worthy of receiving.

This way of being is yours to have. Claim it.

I thrive with the right care for my highly sensitive nature

I was in my early 40s before I realized that I'm a highly sensitive person. I always had a sense that I was different, but I didn't know that it was because my brain was wired differently. According to psychologist Dr Elaine Aron, about 15 to 20 percent of the population is highly sensitive. It's a trait we're born with, and it is a gift to be embraced.

If high sensitivity is a new concept for you, or if you want a recap, here's some info from Psychology Today:

"Highly sensitive people have brains that are structured a little differently from other people. They are wired to absorb more information from the world around them, such as colours, sounds, scents, tastes, and other people's feelings. This is what Elaine Aron calls 'depth of processing,' which is the tendency to process information more deeply. A study by Jadzia Jagiellowicz_found that highly sensitive people use more of the parts of the brain associated with deep processing, especially those that involve noticing subtleties. We absorb information and then we think about it, sorting it, categorising it and comparing it to other things. Sometimes we are aware of this process, but it also happens subconsciously, beneath our awareness, which is why we can feel surprised when we are overwhelmed by all this information we're absorbing."

Many of my favourite people in this whole world are HSWs. I love my non-HSW friends too, but it is with my HSWs that I share the most in common. We are creative and compassionate, we seek deep connection, and we look for meaning in our lives. We can feel what others feel, and we are extremely touched by beauty and love. In a nutshell, we are awesome and have all these special gifts.

I wouldn't trade being an HSW in if I could. It's one of my superpowers. It makes me who I am.

As you know, it's not sunshine and butterflies all the time. HSWs also need special care that others may not. We get easily overwhelmed because of all this processing we do and need more quiet downtime. According to Dr Aron, we're not inherently anxious because we are highly sensitive. We can develop anxiety more easily than others when you compile our sensitive systems with tough childhoods, or difficult life circumstances, or times when there's a lot of bad news out there and people are particularly fearful.

We soak up fear and anxiety like a sponge if we are not careful. We are way more affected by the news. Want to see overwhelm in action? Give an HSW a bad news story and one cup of coffee too much.

I like to think of my highly sensitive nature like being a tree. I'm an awesome tree. I'm not the kind that's going to thrive in parched dirt on the side of a road. I'm more like a poplar or willow – trees that are high-care. I'm choosing to say "high-care" as opposed to "high-maintenance" because that gives an image of a diva on a shopping spree, and that's so far from what an HSW is or needs. Want to see overwhelm in action? Bring an HSW to a mall.

So, my lovely, highly sensitive woman, take the time and space you need to rest, to disconnect from the news, and to reconnect to yourself and to LOVE.

My self talk:

- When I honour my sensitivity, I flourish.
- I give myself permission to get the care I need.
- I take time to mellow out.
- It's ok for me to disconnect from the news and focus on me.
- I may be feeling fear and anxiety that's not even mine. I am just absorbing them like a sponge. I can release this energy and get back to my real nature, to my own real feelings.

A celebration of us

All right. Here's a love letter for you, my dear HSW. It's an ode to all that you are just by being you. It's a celebration of how the world is rendered better because you are in it.

I love that you are so sensitive.

You are wise, so wise. You have knowing.

I love that you feel the truth, even when others try to hide it.

I love how conscientious you are.

I love how good you are.

I love how gifted you are.

I love how intuitive you are.

I love how compassionate you are, even while being strong and powerful and setting boundaries.

I love how you make this world a more thoughtful, quiet, and relaxing place to be.

I love how you can really see me when I'm with you. You really look at me and I know you are present.

I love that when I tell you something, you go away and think about it and may come back to me to talk about it further. You give it consideration.

I love that you respond so well to all kinds of healing modalities.

How wonderful that you are touched so deeply by music, by art, by beauty.

I love the sanctuaries you create in your home, in your studio, in your workplace.

You connect so strongly to nature, to the ocean, to the sun, to the rain, to rocks, to trees, to animals, to soil.

You are a master gardener, encouraging all kinds of life to grow.

You are a peacemaker.

I love how creative you are.

I love how fun you are.

I love how capable of love you are.

I love how you need time alone to come back to yourself, to reflect, to contemplate. This quiet and stillness benefits the whole world.

You are touched and saddened by cruelty and injustice. It is incomprehensible to you that people would act in ways that harm each other.

I love your sense of humour.

I love that you are very careful about what media products you consume.

I love that you use natural products, buy organic and visit farmers markets.

I love that you make food that's wholesome and delicious.

I love that wherever you are, it's a better place than before.

I love that you amend and atone and apologize.

I love that you forgive because you feel so deeply how freeing that is.

I love that we exist. I love how important our role is. I love us.

What do you cherish about being an HSW?

Dear highly sensitive woman, keep your energy high

Yesterday, I asked my 10-year-old daughter to cut my hair. Yes, you read that right, my 10-year-old, whose only experience with scissors thus far was making crafts. In a moment that can only be described as folly, I gave her a pair of professional-grade scissors and asked her to cut a wee bit off the bottom of my hair. Then I sat down and relaxed. First thing I knew, there were long, seven-inch strands of hair on the floor. She understood the directions as "cut mama's hair even," so she chopped off my locks to match the shortest layer. How does it look? Well, like a 10-year-old cut it, but to tell the truth, it's not the worst look I've ever had, it was convenient, and the price was right. It was a lockdown low point, and you may wonder how I got there.

The reason I asked my budding little stylist to give me a cut was that I am doing all that I can to keep my energy and vibration high. As part of that, I've been very aware of who I spend my time with and where I go, and that includes hair salons. As a highly sensitive woman, I take on other people's feelings and energy like a sponge mopping a spill off the counter. We are collectively experiencing loads of fear, anxiety, and anger. That's a huge spill for an HSW to sponge up.

It's crucial that we all take care of ourselves right now. I know my highly sensitive friends are doing what they can to keep their energy high. They are taking long walks, meditating, listening to uplifting music and lectures. They are taking good care of themselves and their loved ones. They keep refuelling themselves. They are doing lots of work feeling their feelings and releasing them as needed. They are also speaking to themselves with as much compassion, patience, and love as they can. They are being HSW-smart.

As the world reopens, we may be feeling some anxiety about it, and wonder if it's really safe. There are many decisions to make about who to see and where to go. Many non-sensitive people are gung-ho to get this party started and kickstart the world back to the way it was before. It's a lot for an HSW to navigate. Again, keeping our energy high will help us sail through the reopening more smoothly.

My intense intention right now is to be as healthy as I can be. I think of it as putting health in my system every day in a myriad of ways. There are the regular suspects, like nourishing foods, lots of water, and early bedtimes, and the practices that make my heart sing, like soulful music and a cup of tea in the morning light. I speak to myself with love and treat myself with kid gloves. This is not the time for perfectionism and self-criticism – not that it ever is. We HSWs learn easily with gentle encouragement and respond beautifully to unconditional approval.

My intense intention is also to take care of my family, my community, and my world in ways that honour who I am as a highly sensitive person. I'm not the best candidate for a large, noisy rally as an HSW, but there are loads of other ways I can contribute and be of service. I can be a warrior for love in a way that's HSW-smart. I can make a significant contribution right now by keeping my energy up. The rising tide raises all boats in the harbor.

I've been staying away from grocery stores during peak hours, public places, Zoom calls with certain groups. This includes some relatives when they are in a particularly bad mood and are looking to have a good dump. You know what I mean by taking a good dump, don't you? It's when a person decides to dump it all on you, like a dump truck unloading trash. They purge their feelings, stress, and anger in a barrage of incessant talking. They walk away feeling lighter, and you slink away carrying their burden. Psychologists call this kind of person an energy vampire, as they suck the life force and energy right out of you. HSWs are particularly yummy to these people. Our empathy makes us targets, as we listen deeply and care.

Navigating the present circumstances of the world doesn't leave me with loads of extra energy. There are activities and people that I just cannot afford. They are just way over my daily energy allowance. The other day, I brought my daughter to a ski resort to go snow tubing as a special treat. It was fun, but loud and way too stimulating. I was so toast after that excursion you could have buttered me right up and served me for breakfast. I kind of limped through the rest of the day and was in bed by 8 pm.

Like a cell phone, I have a certain amount of power until I am done, before I get overwhelmed and am in serious need of recharging. Right now, leading my right life, one in which I am healthy, calm, and at ease, doing my work, and caring for myself and my family, takes most of my daily power. There's not that much left over for extras. Going snow tubing put me in a deficit. It was good fun, and my daughter had a hoot, but the truth is that it came with a price.

You know what I'm talking about here, HSWs, right? It's going to cost something. The question is: Is the price worth it to you? Is it worth saying yes when you mean no? Can you afford to speak with that person right now? Trash TV may be entertaining, but what will it do to your energy reserves? The answer may be yes, that it's worth whatever it costs, but it's good to be aware of the impact it has on you.

On the other end of the spectrum are the people, places, and practices that fill us right up and recharge us. I've been spending as much time as I can in nature and with other HSW kindred souls (mostly on Zoom). If you give me just 20 minutes (the time it takes for an overwhelmed system to calm down) sitting next to a tree outside, I'm a new person. I can spend long moments with my meditation peeps and come out feeling fine, energized, and centered. Having tea with my friend Teresa, a powerhouse of positivity and love, gives me a boost. What about you? What keeps your vibration high?

I think there's no getting around the fact that I'm really going to have to visit the hair salon, but I'm going to do it HSW-smart. I'll make sure it's a small place with few stylists and customers. I'll go first thing in the morning when the energy is high. I'll refuse to engage in gossip with the stylist, or negative talk, because that brings my energy down. I will do all that I can to honor myself and my needs as a highly sensitive woman.

My self talk:

- I honor myself as an HSW.
- I bring great gifts to this world as an HSW.
- I choose the people I spend time with and where I go. There are ways I can be HSW-smart.
- I practice discernment.

The inner DJ

You have a voice inside that's compassion itself, while another is as unforgiving as that ex you broke up with. One voice thinks you're the cat's pyjamas, while the other says you look like something the cat dragged in. Each one of us has the entire spectrum of voices inside. That's just how we are made and wired. Some of the voices speak louder than others and are constantly barraging us with their opinions, while others are gentle, speaking in soft whispers, and you hardly ever hear them.

You can think of these voices like songs on a streaming service. You are the DJ putting the playlist together. You are the one who listens to the music. It's obvious that you are not one of the songs, right? Similarly, you are not the voices you have inside.

We forget we have power, as the DJ, and instead of choosing our music, we stand around numbly, listening to whatever song our brain decides to play for us. We are at its mercy.

My brain used to play me sad songs about how alone I was, or demeaning songs about how I wasn't good enough, or fearful songs about worst-case scenarios. I'd just listen to the music and feel bad, feel low, feel scared, or feel unworthy and small.

It still happens, but now I recognize the tune and I remember who I am – yeah, that's right, the DJ – and I step up and put myself in charge of the music like the quality of my life depends on it – because it does.

I turn one song off, and play a favourite inner song. I instruct the voice of low self-esteem to stop, and ask the voice of unconditional support to play me something sweet. First thing I know, my inner tune sounds like music I enjoy. It makes me want to groove, it makes me feel strong or in love with my life. Some inner songs help me forgive, laugh, calm down, or celebrate. It's the playlist of my own true, good, and brave life.

Don't you want to hear an inner song that makes you jump for joy? Don't you want to hear an inner song that calms you? Don't you want to hear an inner song that makes you feel invincible and propels you to reach for the moon?

They are all there inside you. You may just not be playing them right now.

First thing to know is that you are the DJ. Second thing to know is that, as the DJ, you hold the power to choose the music. And third, you are capable of learning inner DJ skills if need be. So go ahead, start playing the music of your own true, good, and brave life.

My top 5 inner songs:

- I am good enough just the way I am.
- Of course, I can do it.
- I love you.
- It's going to be ok.
- I am here. I will always be with you.

When your wise inner voice says no, but you say yes anyway

What happens to you when your wise inner voice says no, but you overrule it and say yes instead? Where is the line between kindness towards others and disrespecting your own self?

Here's what I mean:

I'm asked to do a favour, and my inner voice says no immediately. I just don't have the resources (time, energy, space, etc.) to say yes to this. Instead, I say yes. I'm regretting it even as I say it, and I'm already starting to resent it.

I'm in the middle of a "conversation" with someone and I realize they are dumping on me. They are releasing a ton of negative thoughts and words all over me. I'm listening to them, wanting to help lift their spirits, and it is coming to the detriment of my own. Suddenly, my inner voice goes, "No, no more. This doesn't feel good at all."

I stay there and keep listening even as I feel myself start to go flat.

This wise inner voice knows what I need and has my highest and greatest good at heart. When it says no, I can trust that it has good reasons. It has no other agenda than my well-being and living an authentic life filled with meaning and goodness. Me, I've got a bunch of other agendas:

I want to help. This is such a chronic response in me. Maybe I over-help? Maybe I'm addicted to helping?

I value kindness and compassion.

I want to save others and resolve their problems. Is this how I give myself value? Like I'm only worthy if I am of help to others…

I want to help them feel better.

I don't trust that they can handle their own business.

I feel sorry for them.

I want to hang on to a relationship, and fear it will come to an end if I say no.

In a way, when I say yes, it's a lie. I'm not giving my real, authentic answer.

I had a wise therapist who said that it was better for your health to choose to say no and feel guilty, than to say yes and feel resentment. (It's that toxic.)

My friend Lori-Ann, who is an awesome composer, author, and spiritual teacher, talks about having reverence for yourself. Reverence is not a word that we use a lot these days. It means holding yourself in high esteem and respect. For me, it means learning to listen to my inner voice as my most trusted guidance. It means standing up for myself with a gentle no, or a more forceful no when it is required. It means enthusiastically saying yes when I know that's my real answer.

My self talk:

- If I say no to someone and they get angry, it doesn't mean I should have said yes.
- If I say no to someone and they don't like me anymore, it doesn't mean I should have said yes.
- I take good care of myself by saying no when it is needed.

- I solidly stand by myself.
- No one needs me to rescue them. They are grown-ups capable of leading their own lives and making their own decisions.
- I can love without over-helping.
- I am free.

She said, I hate myself, and I thought, ouch

We say "I hate myself" without thinking much about it, but part of you takes it very seriously. That part of you wilts under the power of those mean words.

I was at the post office today, mailing copies of my book Speaking to Yourself with Love to a bookstore. The woman working at the counter got all excited when she saw them. "I would like to read it, but I don't read anymore."

She talked about how much she loves reading, and all the lovely books she has, including a collection of spiritual books her mother left her. She no longer takes the time to read. "I'm always on my tablet now," she said. And then she finished with, "I hate myself."

Ouch, I thought. How painful for that part of her that just heard that.

Research shows that every cell in your body hears all that you say. Your body actually listens to what you are saying inside. Your cells hear all your self talk through sound waves and sensory transmissions. They react according to what they hear.

Dr Judith Orloff writes that when we criticize ourselves, it is like an inner war goes on inside us. We turn against ourselves. It is like an attack on our system.

Now think about how your cells rejoice when they hear words of love, acceptance, and compassion.

So just keep putting love into your inner words as much as you can. Step by step, day by day.

We are all just doing our best.

There is no one to hate. There is just someone to love.

My self talk:

- I love myself.
- I am worthy of love.
- I am doing my best.

The inner voice you hear most loudly

No matter how negative, critical, alarming, catastrophizing, or even downright abusive your inner voice may be, you can be sure of one thing: it's not your fault that it sounds like that.

We all have a basic inner voice that pipes up when we are not concentrating on something that takes all our attention. That voice is called the default mode network (DMN). Each person has their own custom DMN, and that voice can range from cruel and abusive all the way to a comforting, loving inner friend. You basically default back to that same voice all the time.

For some people, the DMN is so savage that it is unbearable to spend even a few moments without reaching for a distraction to drown it out. We all have our favourite distractions. I had a long list of them that ranged from working long hours to drinking a lot of wine.

The thing is, once the distraction was gone, my negative self talk was there waiting for me. There was nothing that I could achieve in the outer world, there was no distraction big enough, to change the setting and tone of this inner voice.

It's very stressful to be constantly criticized – even if it's in your own self, done by you. It feels so true when an inner voice is filled with critical, cruel or alarmist words.

I had to go inside to make that change.

There are many different reasons why your own DMN sounds the way it does – none of which are your fault. It's the way your brain is wired for now.

And the wonderful news is that brains can be changed. Neuroplasticity is the ability of your brain to change. If you want to change your inner voice, it is possible. It is in your control to transform your self talk.

The nature of your DMN has nothing to do with whether you're a good person, how accomplished or educated you are, or the contributions you make to this world.

You can be Julia Roberts – with full-on looks, an academy award, a family, fame, and fortune – and still have a savage DMN.

I think Julia Roberts is awesome and I hope she has a gentle and kind DMN – which is something I hope for you too. And if you don't have a compassionate and loving one today, it doesn't mean you won't have one very soon if that's what you choose for yourself. Self Talk Love is a path you can walk – one that leads to more well-being, self-warmth, health, and joy with every kind inner word.

My self talk:

My self talk is in my power.

I can learn loving and positive self talk skills.

I am completely innocent of how my self talk has sounded until now.

I can choose a new path for myself.

You have the power to make your inner self a safehouse

I heard a woman on the radio say she came home from work one day so stressed out and filled with negative self talk that she realized her head was not a safe place for her to be. She sat in the bath and listened to a podcast to drown out her inner voice. She figured it had nothing good to say to her.

Her inner bully was on a rampage, and listening to it for even a few seconds was unbearable. I can understand why she wanted to drown it out. I used to do that all the time. I constantly filled my senses so that I wouldn't hear what my inner voice had to say. It was like a nagging and critical roommate I tried to avoid by staying out late. But she ambushed me. She'd start telling me how I always made mistakes, how I was a fake, how I was underserving and unimportant. It was disheartening. Was I really such a piece of trash that I deserved nothing better than this emotional abuse?

It would have been unthinkable that I would speak to another person the way I spoke to myself. So how was it ok that I said these words to myself? I was anxious from hearing this voice, and from trying to outrun it and block it out. It was not a skilful nor peaceful way to live.

There is so much stress for us to cope with already in this world. If we top that off with inner words that cause more stress, fear, doubt, and putdowns, no wonder so many of us have anxiety. Sometimes our heads are really not a safe place for us to be.

That can be changed.

I was able to make my inner self a safe place to be, a kind of safehouse if you will. It took some work, time, and practice, but it was well worth the effort. There's freedom on the other side, peace of mind, and way more love. I still practice every day to catch myself when needed and speak to myself like all human beings are worthy of: with dignity, forgiveness, kindness, encouragement, and compassion.

Now if I come home from an incredibly stressful day, I want to sit quietly with myself. I want to hear what my inner voice is saying because if it is critical and bullying, I want to manage it.

The thing is, this inner voice, this default inner voice, it doesn't change on its own. It doesn't suddenly one day get better on its own. It needs YOU to decide to transform it from bully to friend, from nasty to kind. It needs YOU to choose a path where there is more love, a sense of worthiness, more joy, and more inner peace.

Today's takeaway is this: it is fully in your power to change your default inner voice. Life comes to meet you when you make a true decision and set your intention. There are so many ways that you can transform your self talk, whether that's self talk transformation exercises, books, professional counselling, meditation, loving kindness practices, or all of the above. The first step is to decide, and to know that you can change if you choose to. You are that powerful.

My self talk:

- I can change.
- I can choose a path with more self-love and inner peace.
- It is possible.
- I am a safe space for myself.

An inner story reset

It all went sideways this morning. For some reason, I thought I had time to bake muffins for my daughter's lunch. What possessed me, I do not know, for on most mornings we barely have time to get the essentials done. At the very last moment I'm waiting for the muffins to be ready, and of course they're not. The soup I was going to put in her thermos was way too spicy and so had to be ditched. I spilled a big bottle of smoothie all over my clothes and the floor. I'm shouting for my husband to get the dog – that canine vacuum – out of the kitchen before he licks it up. The counters are covered in flour, bowls, and food. Finally, I start shoving all kinds of last-minute items into the lunch box as my daughter keeps saying, I have to go, I have to go.

The stakes were low on this, yet I was feeling frazzled by the chaos and by the rush. I completely overextended myself for no good reason. I got a little worked up and so did my inner critic. When I get stressed and anxious, negative self talk starts. This is normal. Stress and my inner critic are old buddies. When one shows up, the other one   isn't   far   behind.

If I don't do something about it, they tend to work each other up. The self talk gets more negative, and that makes me feel more anxious. I feel more stress and the inner words get more critical. I'm stuck in a loop.

This has happened to me in all kinds of situations, from meetings where I thought I said the so-called wrong thing, to having to deal   with   emergencies.

I realized I needed a self talk reset. I needed to reset my energy and my self talk. I needed to stop this frazzled feeling and step back into a calm power. If not, it would have a snowball effect that would build momentum all day. I needed to take a pause to allow myself this self talk reset. It doesn't   take   very   long.

I took a few deep breaths right into my heart center. I made my mind quieter. I made my heart more open. I told myself about   what   I   was   feeling.

Then I re-positioned the morning's story. I gave it another angle. Instead of being upset by the mess I made of it, I told myself funny things about it. (It must have been quite the sight!) I also told myself about what I'm grateful for. Levity and gratitude are two of the best ways I know to reset. I recentered myself and brought my energy back to me. I had a self talk reset.

A self talk reset can be helpful for life's stressful little moments like this morning. It can also be a game-changer when there's a bigger concern going on. It's made a difference to me in much more stressful situations, like the emergency ward at the hospital.

Here are the steps to a self talk reset:

- Step 1: Take some time and space for the reset.

- Step 2: Stop the momentum of stressful, negative self talk with deep breaths, quieting the mind, and opening the heart.

- Step 3: Tell yourself about your feelings regarding the situation. It will help you have clarity. It will also help you relax when you realize you have been seen and heard.

- Step 4: Give the story a new angle and change your inner words about it. Can you find something comical or something that makes you grateful about it? Tell yourself all about it.

- Step 5: Repeat as needed. Keep showing up and being your own leader, stepping towards more inner words of love and calm.

My self talk:

- I can use my inner words to have more inner calm and love.
- I can do a self talk reset anytime.
- My inner words are safe and loving.

4 favorite ways to stop negative self talk

When my self talk is filled with criticism, recriminations, anxious fears, regrets, and putdowns that go on and on, I turn to these tried-and-true techniques to get a break from the inner critic.

1.You have the power to switch it off

If you are playing a negative story in your head, switch it off just like you would turn off a song that you don't like. Simply imagine pressing the off button. If the song starts again, press the off button again. Switch it off as many times as you need to. Remember that you are in charge here. You get to decide what words you tell yourself.

It's your job to protect yourself from any voice inside that mistreats you. No one else is inside you and can do this for you. You must play the role of superhero protector

47

for yourself. By pressing the off button, you are standing up for yourself and saying, "Stop it. Enough already. Give me a break with your criticism and negative self talk."

2. Specifically focus on something positive

When you catch yourself in a downward spiral of negative self talk, bring your focus to something or someone that is incredibly positive for you. For example, if I'm stuck in a loop of thinking about a conflict, I will bring my attention to someone whom I love and get along with really well. I'll tell myself about my grandmother or my meditation teacher, or a favourite holiday destination, or the yellow and purple tulips in my garden that make me smile.

3. Tone down the catastrophizing

Catastrophizing is when you tell yourself that the worst will happen or make a way bigger deal out of a situation than it is. My friend once gave herself back spasms imagining worst-case scenarios about her new job.

You can tone down the inner conversation by sticking with the details of a situation or using words that are not so charged. For example, instead of telling yourself that "it's a disaster" when there's a leak in the ceiling, tell yourself, "there's a leak in the ceiling and it will be fixed as soon as possible." Instead of saying "my life sucks," tone it down to "I had a difficult day at work. I'm going to rest now and recharge."

4. Gratitude

Focus on what you do have, and the good in your life. You get to decide if you want to tell yourself about the abundance in your life or the lack of what you don't have. I know a spiritual teacher who has worked with several billionaires who feel like they still don't have enough money. Believing that you live in abundance is a state of being. Tons of studies show that a gratitude practice makes you feel better about yourself and about your life. Tell yourself a few things you are thankful for every day, or write them down. Who knows how it will change your life to immerse yourself in the good.

Nighty night to a chatterbox mind

I make it a priority to cultivate a quiet mind. As an HSW, I really need the peace that a quiet mind gives me. I find it hard to fall asleep if my mind is swirling.

Sometimes when I go to bed, my mind races. I don't even notice. I get totally caught up in the emotions of it. A train of thought comes by, and I jump right onto it. The first thing I know, I've ridden this train all the way across the continent to New York. I am not even noticing anymore that I am safely and quietly in bed. In my head, I'm entangled in some kind of problem or situation. The moment I notice, though, the moment I catch it, its time is numbered.

That's because I know that a racing mind at bedtime – analyzing myself, judging myself, other people, or situations – doesn't have a happy ending. It doesn't enable my already tired nervous system to calm down. It doesn't enable me to rest and rejuvenate. I will take measures immediately to calm it down. I'll repeat the measures again and again until my mind settles, like mud at the bottom of a lake.

This modern world is quite taxing. Our energy and attention are pulled into all kinds of directions and situations. You are not going to find a solution to anything at bedtime by analyzing something until your mind is completely frazzled by it. You've made it through another day. Well done, you! Your gift now is that you get to rest. Highly sensitive women need more sleep than the average person. Our nervous system is more vigilant and needs this longer restoration. A good night's sleep enables us to be ready to live the 16 hours of our day when we are awake.

Here are a few tricks I use when I catch myself in the act of analyzing or fretting or judging at bedtime.

The other night, I started down the road of "why did this... and why did that..." Then I gave up. I said to myself: "You did your best. That's all."

- The switcheroo: If I catch myself in negative self talk about anything, I will immediately change my inner words to some that are positive and loving. If I'm going to tell myself stories about anything, it might as well be about things and people that bring me joy and make me feel love.

- The metal box: If I catch myself going over a problem, I'll imagine putting it in a big, solid metal box and securing a lid to it. Then this metal box is put into a warehouse that has millions of similar metal boxes lined up on shelves. (Think of how they hid the ark in Raiders of the Lost Ark.) The situation can wait for me over there.

- Attention in my feet: I'll put my attention as far away from my head as possible. I'll bring my awareness to my feet and keep it there. I'll just feel my feet.

Wishing you good rest and a peaceful mind.

My self talk:

- I have earned a good night's sleep.
- I take good care of myself in the evening and help myself relax.
- All can wait. This is my time to rest.

It may have nothing to do with you – the energy that surrounds us

As an HSW, I am capable of picking up on the energy that surrounds me. I can sense the energy walking into a room or while having a conversation with someone. We communicate so much energetically, just with our presence. Your body picks up on it, a kind of somatic intelligence. Your intuition picks up on it.

We are all connected and share a collective energy. Each one of us adds to the shared energy, and we receive what others put in it. It's like we are all in the same ocean sharing a body of water. You'd be affected by anyone who polluted the water and, conversely, by anyone who made a positive contribution by making the water cleaner and healthier.

There are people and places that elevate us. Their energy vibrates high and we leave their presence feeling calm, good, joyous. I've had experiences being in large groups of people meditating and opening their hearts where I was absolutely elevated by the energy. I felt terrific and in love with all of life.

I've had the opposite experience of being deflated, anxious, or tired after an encounter with one person or in a group setting. In fact, it's very rare that I don't feel overwhelmed after being in a group.

How you feel after seeing someone is a good indicator of what's really going on beneath the surface. You can't always put your finger on the reason why you feel that way, but it is real. I want to validate the sensation. You are not making it up. You may never know why being with a person makes you feel that way. It is real and it is true. You don't need anyone else to notice or to feel the same way. This is one of our many HSW gifts – we feel these things.

For instance, I may leave somewhere and feel angry, anxious, or a little depressed. After I have a sudden change in my mood or energy level, I'll ask myself: Is this mine? Sometimes I can actually feel that something isn't mine. It is an energy that I have picked up or am sensing.

Each of us emanates an electromagnetic field. The love we feel inside radiates out of us. The anxiety we feel radiates out of us too. Each of my inner words carries an energy that I feel and that radiates out of me. It's important that I choose my inner words carefully. In her book Power Words, Sharon Anne Klingler writes that words "carry their own power and are an integral part of your electromagnetic field."

We also have a collective energy field around our planet. There is a geomagnetic field that surrounds the Earth that's called the Schumann Resonance. It's been called the heartbeat of the Earth and has been measured since the 1950s. On April 4, 2020, a global meditation was organized online. Hundreds of thousands of people meditated at the same time. That day, the Schumann Resonance jumped to the point of 76, the highest that it's ever been recorded.

This is just one example of the collective energy that we share together. As HSWs, we tend to feel energy deeply. It's our very own guidance system. We know when something or someone is right for us. And we know when we need to take leave as soon as we possibly can.

My self talk:

- I trust the energy that I feel.
- I don't need to know why the energy is a certain way to be able to read it.
- Being able to feel energy is one of my gifts as an HSW.
- I can ask myself: Is this mine?

My soul belongs to me

I am free. I am a sovereign person, and as such, I get to decide what anything means to me, and what I accept as true. I have boundless power.

I have complete freedom over the following and way more:

- I get to decide the meaning a situation has for me.
- I get to decide what my self talk is, and what I will accept in my inner speech.
- I get to decide what words I use to describe myself, my life, and those around me.
- I get to decide who I am.
- I get to decide what I say about who I am.
- I get to decide if I open my heart and open my mind.
- I get to decide if I have faith and what that looks like.
- I get to decide what I will not participate in and with my participation make stronger — things

like fear, gossip, criticism, judging and shaming.

- I get to decide how I care for my inner self and my body.
- I get to decide what I say.
- I get to decide how I act.
- I get to decide what love I will give and to whom.
- I get to decide whether something is a yes or a no for me.
- I get to decide what is important to me, and how to live in accordance with that.

My soul is my own. It cannot be bought, coerced, or stolen. My soul belongs to me.

My self talk:

- I am free.
- My soul belongs to me.
- I decide what meaning I give everything and everyone in my life.
- I choose to open my heart and open my mind.

What a badass Maasai woman taught me about self talk

My friend Ruth travelled to Africa and brought back for me a colourful beaded necklace made by a Maasai woman. It's stunning and you can wrap it around your neck like a scarf, it's so long.

Ruth said she knew the necklace was mine as soon as the Maasai woman started speaking to her. She told Ruth the necklaces she makes and sells are a solid financial contribution to her tribe. Others, especially the men, may talk a big game about what they do and how important they are, but she – quietly and solidly – knows the value of who she is and what she does. She doesn't need anyone to tell her or acknowledge it.

Sometimes, I find myself waiting for acknowledgement. Or a pat on the back. Or for someone to notice what I'm doing – or who I am.

An outside validation – while nice – is never going to change how I feel inside. That's entirely up to me.

Ruth is always saying that I've inspired her to change her self talk, but now, she – and that badass Maasai woman – have inspired me.

I'm not waiting for someone to give me flowers. I'm planting my own garden. I can use my positive and loving self talk to remind myself of who I am and how precious my life is.

My self talk:

- I know who I am.
- I know who I am.
- I know who I am.
- I know what I contribute.
- I know what I know.
- I know my value to myself, to my family, to my friends, to my community.
- I am worthy.

The inner voice of kindness

I was on a group call on Zoom recently when a woman mentioned that she was taking this time to eat a crazy healthy diet and had already lost 4 pounds – on her butt. Then she said she had a big backside and had really needed to lose that weight.

I'm all for nutritious eating. Anything that we can do to stay healthy, strong, and robust is vitally important. Butt, can we give our rusty dusty – our whole bodies, for that matter – a break for now? Or maybe forever?

No one needs more stress right now. What we all need is to be treated with kid gloves. It matters what you say to yourself. Part of you is listening to everything you say and reacts in the same way it would if someone else said those cruel words. In addition, every cell in your body "hears" what you say. It gets a message that either elevates it or brings it down. When your cells hear kind, happy messages, they rejoice and can work optimally.

Many research projects have shown that kindness is an incredible boost to the immune system. Dr David Hamilton, a researcher and author of many books on the health benefits of kindness, writes: "In a number of different ways, kindness produces opposite effects from those that stress causes."

Right at this moment, we are all in need of extreme kindness. We need someone to show us compassion, patience, and support and to be there for us. That someone is you. Your own self-kindness can be a game-changer.

Think of someone who is truly kind to you. How does that person speak to you? Now you've got a model. I think of my friend Leslie.

The other day, again on Zoom, I told Leslie about a lie I told. I was quite ashamed about it. I've been striving to be authentic and live with integrity, and I came up short. "Oh hon…" she said. She looked at me with so much kindness and told me that I was just human. This brought me such comfort. She didn't judge me. She loves me just as I am – strengths and flaws and all. What a gift!

I want to treat myself, to speak to myself, the way Leslie treats and speaks to me. I, too, can be at ease with the fact that I am a human who makes mistakes. How much lighter will I feel in embracing all of me with kindness?

We can be that way with ourselves: show extreme kindness. What kind words can you say to yourself? Your body will love it, your spirit will love it, your mind will love it too.

My self talk:

- I love you the way you are.
- You don't have to be perfect for me to love you.
- How are you? What do you need right now?
- I see you.
- I am right here.
- I forgive you.
- I am giving myself the benefit of the doubt.
- You don't need any additional stress right now.
- I'm going to treat you with kid gloves.

The voice is self-protection – standing up for yourself

My cousin Caroline is a psychologist who worked for years in the court system with children who had been abused. She once told me that the children who were the most hurt were not necessarily the ones who had suffered the most abuse. The children who were the most wounded were the ones whose moms knew of the abuse and ignored it. The mothers hadn't stood up to protect the children.

It's very powerful when someone stands up for you. You feel supported, elevated, protected, loved. You feel like you matter. It also makes you feel like you are not alone.

If your self talk is cruel, critical, or even verbally abusive, it's in your power to do something about it. You can be that person who stands up for yourself. You can make a difference in your life by standing up for yourself and offering protection from your own self.

Neuroimaging shows that part of your brain listens to everything that the other part says. It's like you are having a conversation with yourself. Imagine the toll that it takes on you to be listening to an inner speech that is filled with cruelty.

So, take notice. What are you saying to yourself? Here are some of the words that my inner bully has said to me:

- Who do you think you are?
- There is something wrong with you.
- You can't count on anyone else.
- You will always be alone.
- You are unlovable.
- You are a fraud.
- You mess everything up.
- It's always your fault.
- You look terrible.
- You are a bad person.

Verbal abuse is detrimental wherever it comes from – including self-generated. Once I noticed how I spoke to myself, I was able to do something about it. I choose to do something about it.

You have the power to stand up to that negative, abusive voice and protect yourself. You can be that person for yourself. You can be the person you have been waiting for all those years. You can speak to yourself like a real best friend or a loving parent would.

What you say to yourself internally today will plant the seeds for how you are, and how you live tomorrow.

When I first began this journey of loving self talk 15 years ago, it was such a new concept for me to consider that what I said to myself could have an impact on me and my life.

Just like how water shapes rock over time, we are shaped with what we hear every day and how that makes us feel. Our brain is shaped by what it hears. Our cells are shaped by what they hear.

Every time that we say a kind word to ourselves, every time we turn towards ourselves with warmth, compassion, and love, it counts. It accumulates and then it gets easier to do. The inner loving words are small and the stuff of everyday life, but they are powerful over time.

I tell my daughter that a lot of life happens step by step, with every decision, with every practice, with every kind inner word. It's the stuff of everyday life.

Sometimes, we need help finding a path that's meaningful and loving, but once we are on it, it's up to us to put one foot in front of the other. Many teachers have pointed me in the right direction and given me tools, but I am the one who decides every day how I want to treat myself.

I speak to myself differently now, for the most part. I still fall back on my default mode of negative, critical self talk sometimes, especially when I'm over-tired, anxious, or having a conflict with someone. I may then attack myself inside with cruel or dismissing words that make me feel small. Thankfully, it doesn't last too long now. I hear it. I catch it. And then I speak tender words to myself because of what I just went through: I was hurt by my own inner words. Then once again, I choose inner words of love and compassion. Step by step like water on stone.

My self talk:

- You are important to me.
- You deserve that I take good care of you.
- You are doing your absolute best.
- I love you just the way you are.

The gentleness of taking the time we need for healing

When your mind, body, or spirit are showing signs of needing rest, care, or healing, stop and take the time that's needed. In your self talk, you can give yourself permission to do so.

Think of it like getting a flat tire.

If you were driving down the street and you suddenly got a flat tire, would you keep driving? You would stop and take care of what needs taking care of. You would do that no matter what you had planned that day. You would do that no matter what commitments were hanging over your head. You would put all else on hold while you dealt with what needed to be dealt with – even if it were highly inconvenient.

Now, what could happen if you didn't pull over to fix the tire? It could lead to a bunch of problems much worse and more dangerous than a flat tire. You could damage the car. You could lose control of the vehicle. You could hurt yourself, or even kill yourself, or the individuals unlucky enough to be in your way.

Well, that is how it can be with self-care. When your mind, body, or spirit are suffering from a flat tire, you can tend to it without delay. Taking the time you need to heal yourself is preventative. Unless you want to move on to a more dangerous and damaging situation, you really have no choice. When your health and well-being are at stake, you slow down your life and take care of yourself. You do that because you are wise. You do that because it's an act of love and mercy.

"I have come to believe that caring for myself is not self-indulgent. Caring for myself is an act of survival." – Audre Lorde

My self talk:

- I take good care of myself.
- I am worthy of self-care.
- I take all the time that I need to nurture my health and well-being.
- I just don't have the resources to do everything that I used to do. Right now, I need to care for myself.
- I know I had other plans, but this is what is needed today.

Trusting the signs that life gives you

This morning my dog, who loves to walk in the forest like all dogs, refused to go in. I tried to pull him along about 20 times, but he kept sitting and refusing to walk. Very strange indeed.

Then my intuition kicked in and I suddenly wondered if he knows something that I don't. Does he smell something? Does he feel something? A danger, a bear, a cougar?

I turned around. Despite my disappointment because I had gone out of my way to hike in this forest, I had to trust. There must be a reason that I have no business in this forest this morning.

I believe that life gives me signs and that it's up to me if I want to follow them. As strange as some of them have been, they have never let me down.

When I got back in the car, a French song about trusting yourself strongly was playing on the radio.

Trust.

That's my word for today. What does it look like to trust myself? What does it look like to trust my life and the signs it gives me?

It's so hard to trust. It's hard to trust that everything is going to be ok. It's so hard to not try to control everything, even if I know that doesn't work and it is completely exhausting to live that way. It's so hard to relax and to not be at attention, hyper-vigilant, on the lookout for problems and danger.

There was a time when I would have needed a much stronger sign than a dog refusing to walk. I would have needed a bunch of signs that would have escalated in urgency until I had no choice but to follow them.

I'll never know for sure if I was right to turn around this morning, but I have less of a need to know. I decided to trust, and that's all there is to it. I know that life's signs point the way like a lighthouse. I can trust them and myself to make decisions based on them.

And when I say inside: I trust myself, I trust life, I trust the divine, I can feel my whole body relax.

My self talk:

- I trust.
- I trust the signs that life gives me. They are the arrows pointing the way, they are the steppingstones.
- I trust the decisions that I make.
- I trust that when I make mistakes, I will learn from them and move on.
- I trust my life.
- I trust the divine.
- I trust myself.

Setting an intention and following the steps to a new life

You may think that progress in life is made in huge leaps – and you are right. Suddenly an idea comes, a solution appears, an intention is set, a miracle happens. Moving forward also involves a series of small steps, one in front of the other. Over time they build up, giving momentum to a new course.

Let me give you an example. I suffered from chronic pain in my shoulder blade for several years. It was constantly flaring up. I had seen all kinds of healers and practitioners, but I had come to believe that this is just something I had to live with, that all I could do was to take the edge off it.

Just over one year ago, I set the intention that I was going to find a solution to it. I had to trust that it was possible, and to tell myself that it was possible. I found a new team of sports injury practitioners who were able to diagnose what I had and give me a treatment plan. Then, every day since then, I have been doing the exercises and stretches that they gave me.

Now I am free of pain, and my overall posture is much more solid. The great leap was the intention, the trust, and finding a new team. The step-by-step has been doing those exercises every day – as boring as it is.

There is such power in showing up regularly and doing the work – whatever that is. With your self talk you can encourage yourself to show up, to keep going, and to believe in what you are doing. Of course, you've got to be headed in the right direction. You can walk step-by-step towards a sunset, but if you are facing the wrong way, you'll never see one. And when we realize we're not headed where we want to go, then we change course. We are always allowed to set the course for our right life.

We may become unsure of the direction or the next step. We may be in the dark about it. We may need to pause. We pause and contemplate. We pause and seek information. We pause and check in with our inner self. We pause and read the signs that show themselves to us. We pause and let the answer come. Sometimes, information only comes at the very last moment. You can't force it. You may only become clear on the very next step that can be taken.

We may feel anxious about not knowing. How we want to know it all and control it all. We think that's how we are safe. A feeling of deep safety only comes when we are able to trust that it's all going to work out and that we will know the next step when the time comes.

You trust that the step after that will be illuminated for you. It's just like when you drive at night. You can only see a limited distance ahead of you, but you know that as you move forward, more of the road will be visible. You are wise, and you know that when it is very dark and the road is treacherous, you must drive very slowly. This is where trust comes in. To trust that when the moment is right, what you need to see will be illuminated. You will know the direction or the next step. You will know what to do, where to go, what to say. And that can mean to do nothing, say nothing, go nowhere, but to stay still for the present moment.

My self talk:

- I trust that I will know when the time is right.
- Step by step, I create my right life.
- It is ok for me to pause when I am not sure and wait for guidance.
- I am allowed to change direction in my life.
- I show up for myself and do the work step by step.

Pat yourself on the back for the endurance you have shown

We can respect the endurance that has been required of us as HSWs. We can salute ourselves for the endurance needed to show up, and to keep loving. That takes endurance.

And what about the endurance needed for all those groundhog days? Chop wood. Carry water. Chop wood. Carry Water. And repeat, repeat, repeat. Get done what needs to get done that moment, that day.

And what about the courage we have shown? And how we've had to dig deep within ourselves to find strength, and faith, and trust?

And what about the resilience we have shown?

And what about the compassion we have shown ourselves and others, and the forgiveness we have given?

And what about the optimism we have shown?

Yes, we are truly worthy of respect for the endurance that we have shown. We have done our best. We have been very capable. We can salute ourselves for that. Big pat on the back. Well done, you!

Keep going, beautiful one. You are more powerful than you know. You are more resilient than you know. You can keep going, caring for yourself and your loved ones. You can keep making this world a more just, caring, and compassionate place. Of course, you can do it. And reach out for help if you need it. Resiliency doesn't mean doing it all alone. It means that you keep going even when it's hard. And if you can also remember all that you have to be thankful for, it will elevate your heart. Keep going. Cheer yourself on. You are   loved.

My self talk:

- I am resilient and strong.
- I am capable.
- I am courageous.
- I keep going step by step, moment by moment, day by day.

- I am powerful beyond belief.
- Thank you for .... and ....
- I am so thankful to be alive.
- It is possible.

Self talk can be like a big, scruffy mutt that needs a good romp

Sometimes it's easy to turn my self talk around. I can calm down a voice of blame or criticism with a gentle reminder of "now, now, enough now, settle down." At other times, well… let's just say that it's as hard as getting a wild dog on a rampage to obey a gentle command.

Sometimes my mind is like a huge dog out of control, grabbing the steaks off the counter, threatening the neighbors with her growls, or running down the block after the mail carrier. For some moments – or, let's face it, for some hours – on tough days, I forget who the master is, and the dog runs rampant, howling, while I am frozen, listening to it, at its mercy.

And then I remember I have a choice in all this. I'm the one who's listening to this howling dog, and frankly, I don't have to. I am the master and it's important for both of us that I step up and act like one. Every dog needs a consistent, boundary-setting, calm, confident, loving, kind master, as Cesar Millan might say. We need to be that kind of master with ourselves, with our inner voices.

As I can choose to learn dog training skills, I can choose to learn positive and loving self talk skills.

One skill that I use when my inner critic needs a good calming down is to move. Movement unblocks an energy within us and permits a softer, kinder inner voice to emerge. This kind voice is always within, but who can hear it under the thunder of an inner critic gone wild? Movement calms the nervous system as well, which in turn calms negative self talk.

Runners say that a good run clears their mind. That's what I'm talking about here. For me, a good swim, dancing alone or in a group, a walk in the woods or on the beach, or a good stretch enables me to let energy go and flow. I can then start speaking to myself kindly and with patience once again. You will also find me punching pillows or screaming underwater as I swim when I really need to get some energy out.

Just like that big old scruffy mutt needs a good romp to let out nervous energy, I also need to move. Then, with more calm, I can hear that loving voice inside who knows that I am awesome as I am.

My self talk:
- I am the master of my self talk.
- I am kind to myself.
- Movement helps me speak kindly to myself.
- I love you.
- What you say inside matters, love.

Blooming into yourself

"And the day came when the risk to remain tight in a bud was more painful than the risk it took to blossom." This is one of my favorite quotes, and it's by Anais Nin – a woman who spoke in her authentic voice in a time that was even harder to do so than now.

It takes some courage to live as you truly are and speak with your own authentic voice. For many years, I kept this true voice of mine under wraps. In my professional life, I worked in PR and wrote and spoke on behalf of my clients, using their voice. In my personal life, I rarely spoke out about my own beliefs and truths. Being agreeable and being so-called "nice" had a higher priority than being me. It was not my original idea to be this way. Pressure was put on me to keep my mouth shut and toe the line, and I was shamed when I didn't play along. After a while, I didn't know anymore what was mine and what wasn't. My own voice was hiding so deep within me that I didn't really know what it sounded like or what it had to say.

It takes a lot of nervous energy to stay hidden and to quell a voice that wants to tell the truth. Not living in accordance with one's truth keeps one on edge. How can you relax when you are not living truly, when you are in fear of discovery?

And yet, there are so many reasons why we feel that we are safer when we keep our mouths shut. History is filled with women who paid an exceedingly high price to be themselves and to tell their truth. We've inherited those genes that say: "Stay small, stay quiet, don't rock any boat, stay alive. What you feel and want and know is not important. Pretend you don't know what you know, and that way, you'll keep the peace and stay safe. Better to betray yourself than to make others around you uncomfortable, angry, or reject you."

I am now coming into my own, finding my true voice. This has happened later in life, and that's ok. In fact, considering that I came from many generations of women who didn't have a voice, it's a great leap forward that I now do have my own true voice.

It takes some courage to take the risk to blossom, as Anais wrote. It is way riskier to stay tight, enclosed in yourself, living a life that doesn't feel right. The process of embodying your own true voice starts inside with self talk. I began by admitting to myself who I was and what I believed. My inner words guide me.

The Buddhists say that we don't really transform; We realize who we really are. It's like taking mud off your windshield, and suddenly you can see. You have a deep knowing of how powerful, good, beautiful, and awesome beyond belief you really are.

What an empowered way for a highly sensitive woman to live when she finds her voice and starts using it – even if doing so goes against all that her family and society told her to be.

"I stopped asking the question of whether or not something I do is good enough, and I started asking 'Is it me enough.'" – Brittney Spencer

My self talk:

- I want to know who I am.
- I want to know what my truth is.
- It is safe to be me.
- I can only be me.
- I was born to be me.

When we tell the truth and stop hiding

I salute all brave, sensitive women who are shedding their masks. They are showing up bare-faced as who they really are and speaking their truths.

I have two highly sensitive friends who are showing up courageously as themselves right now. Both are doing work to go deep inside to discover their true nature and heal. As they go inside, they are feeling way more love for themselves and others. This is spurting their transformation. And as that happens, they feel more power, more strength. They feel the truth of who they are.

As Oprah writes: "What I know for sure is that speaking your truth is the most powerful tool we all have."

These women are waking up to how awesome they are, how much power they have inside. They have begun standing up for themselves, as well as for others. They are speaking out for justice, for human rights, for women's full equality and empowerment.

Sometimes they say things that are just so courageous and wise that I am in awe. Wow, I think, look at that woman go!

This is what my two friends stop doing as they stop wearing masks:

- They stop dimming their own light to stay safe and not be noticed.
- They stop hiding who they really are.
- They stop pretending to be someone else so they will fit in.
- They stop preferring to keep the peace instead of following what is their truth and wisdom.

It can be scary to tell the truth, and it's not always welcomed by those around us. In fact, it makes some people very uncomfortable, and sometimes frightened and angry. Shedding your mask may unbalance the status quo of some of your relationships. Some people around you may benefit from your invisibility and silence, and don't want that to change.

What kind of life is it to keep your beautiful face hidden behind a mask? What kind of life is it to keep your beautiful and true words hidden inside you?

Some women, our Sisters, cannot safely tell the truth. They live inside a home, or in a country, where it is dangerous to do so. For us who can, we can learn to shed our masks for ourselves and for them.

Only you can sing the song you were born to sing. And the world so desperately needs to hear your beautiful song.

My self talk:

- I give myself permission to be me.
- I give myself permission to be vulnerable and say my truth.
- I live truly as my most magnificent, most courageous self.
- Only I can sing this song. Only I can give these gifts.
- I am free.

What brings you joy?

I asked my friend yesterday what first attracted her to her fiancé. She said that he asked her what brings her joy. No wonder she fell for him.

Now I ask you too: what brings you joy?

Why do I ask? Because when you identify what brings you joy, and you start to focus on it in your self talk, it puts positive thinking into your brain.

Our brains are designed with an inclination towards negativity. We are built to take more notice of what's negative. Our brains evolved that way to keep us out of danger. Your brain is more interested in negative self talk.

So it takes lots of small positive inner messages to tip the scales towards more happiness, more joy, more health.

An easy way to get a positive inner message is to focus on what brings you joy. Telling yourself about what brings you joy and fully focusing on it helps tip the scales favourably.

Right now, it's easy for me to do that because everywhere I look I see what brings me joy: spring. Spring's explosive revival of new life, light, and colour buoys me, elevates me.

I use spring to tip my scales towards well-being. Instead of walking quickly by and only giving it a little of my attention, I stand under the cherry blossoms, or in front of the gardens filled with colourful tulips. I let myself feel amazed. I let myself feel grateful for this abundance, for this vibrancy.

I tell myself about it:

- These are so beautiful. I love looking at them.
- I am taking the time to do something I enjoy.
- How lovely to just stand here.
- How lucky I am that it is spring, and my neighbourhood is filled with flowers.
- Look at those trees with all their blossoms. I love them so much!

When something pleases you, absorb it. Let the part of your brain that listens get a big old dose of it.

It really does count. It counts for your health. It counts for your well-being. It counts for your optimism. It counts for your calmness.

What brings you joy that you can spend time today focusing on?

My self talk:

- I pursue what brings me joy with vigour and purpose.
- I take time with the beauty and goodness that surround me.
- I tip the scales towards more happiness and joy.

Awakening to the beautiful in me and all around me

I recently posted a photo of my daughter and me on Facebook. It was for a post I wrote about healing and meditation. Frankly, I look strange in it. I have no makeup and my face is funny. I selected it because you can really see the love that my daughter and I have for each other in it. You can sense the energy. We have our arms around each other, and my daughter's eyes are closed in bliss. I decided that the natural and radiant face of a grown-up woman who loves her daughter is beautiful. Not by the standards of fashion magazines, the cosmetic industry, or pop stars. By my standards. Really, truly, deeply beautiful. How can love be anything else but beautiful?

I was so in love with my grandmother. She was in her 80s, and I thought she was gorgeous with her short blond perm, her pink lipstick, her lined freckled face, and her green eyes. When I love, I see beauty. How can I see anything else?

When we look into the mirror, there is a part of us that comes to life and that gets very excited to see us. "There I am," it says. "Hello!" It reacts just like you would if you suddenly saw a dear friend you hadn't seen in a while. "Hello you!!! OMG so good to see you!"

Now imagine if this dear friend responded like this: "You look awfully tired. Look at those bags under your eyes. Those jeans look tight. Are those new wrinkles on your face?"

You would be crestfallen. This little innocent voice inside that is so happy to see you in the mirror feels the same way.

I can be harsher on myself than I was on my grandmother. When I look in the mirror, I don't only see sunshine and wild roses. My voice of judgement comes up at times. It used to come up every day, but now only makes an occasional appearance, like a guest on a talk show. When it does pop up, I counterbalance it with my other, more loving and accepting voices. I will greet myself. I will tell myself I am beautiful. I will spend a few moments connecting with myself and looking into my own eyes. I'll even sometimes apologize for the criticism or insult.

And the innocent little voice inside beams. She just loves it. She soaks it right up. She is starting to believe me now because she's been hearing this message that I am beautiful for a few years now. What you hear again and again sinks in, and you start to believe it.

As I love myself more, I find myself more beautiful. Because love is beautiful. It cannot be otherwise. My inner words carry the power to open a gateway to self-love and to the belief that I am beautiful just the way I am. Think inner beauty. Think self talk filled with beautiful words.

My self talk:

- You look so beautiful.
- Look at you, you gorgeous woman.
- I am so happy to see you.
- I get to decide what is beautiful.
- I can give that gift to myself.

Honoring the awesomeness of my vagina

Speaking of beauty… I just finished reading the Vagina Bible, and woman – did it ever open my eyes. Our collective internal dialogue on the subject of this sacred body part is less than rosy – pun intended. Our self talk tends to be negative and highly critical of our vaginas. Poor little kitties…

Why is there a contemplation on the vagina in this book? I'll tell you why: If we are not at ease with this essential part of being a woman, how can we be calm in our bodies?

We have been told many ridiculous untruths about our vaginas. It would be hilarious were it not for the fact that we've taken it on and believed it. Men have told us – and last time I checked, they didn't have female genitalia and therefore have no way of knowing – that our vaginas are:

- Too tight
- Too loose
- Too dry

- Too wet – anyone who complains of that has obviously never encountered a vagina having a good time
- Too long
- Too smelly

Make no mistake, a lot of people get power and make a lot of money off women feeling insecure about being women. Corporations push women to buy all kinds of products for "cleanliness" and "odour," which all suck for our health.

Your yoni is one of the essences of being a woman. It is your center of female creative power – and I'm not just talking about baby-making. It is from this sacred centre (which, by the way, corresponds with our first chakra) that power and creativity emerge.

Not being pro-your-own-vagina is like a tree being critical of its leaves, or a flower debasing its petals, or a dog not liking its tail, or a man not thinking his penis is the greatest thing since sliced bread.

The very essence of being a woman cannot be defined by patriarchy or corporate greed. A radical act of self-love? Love your vagina. Say no to the forces that gain when you feel bad about it. Say yes to yourself.

And another thing: This fad of getting rid of all pubic hair? It comes from porn. So much porn is now available that we have adopted its customs into the mainstream. That's crazy on many levels, and really too bad because pubic hair helps protect the vagina and increases female sexual pleasure.

My self talk:

- My vagina is awesome.
- I take good care of my vagina.
- I am proud and delighted to be a woman.
- I decide what my vagina means to me.

Focusing on what we want

It's really easy for us to focus on what we don't want in life. We have inner voices who are wired to do just that. These voices focus on the outcomes that we are trying to avoid, or the things we don't want to see in this world, like:

I don't want to do this job (Ok, so what do you want to do?)

I don't want to live like this anymore (Awesome realization, and now what? What can your life be like?)

I don't want to be alone (Good job! How do you see sharing your life with someone else? What can it look like? How can it be fun? How can it be loving? And meaningful?)

I don't want to feel anxious (Don't we all! What is your intention on how you want to feel?)

It's in your power to guide yourself with your inner words to go towards what you want, like a flower that leans towards the sun.

Think of it like a taxi. Imagine you sit in a taxi and you tell the driver: I don't want to go downtown. And then you say: Don't take me to the mountains either. And then you say: Don't drive me anywhere near Shirley's house. So what's the taxi driver to do? How can they drive you to where you really want to go if there are no instructions, if there is no desired destination?

Not wanting something is a starting point, it's a point of realization. It's very worthwhile because it brings something to your consciousness, like "I don't want my relationship to be like this anymore," or "I don't want to feel so big and heavy in my body." The inner voice of discontent has brought something legitimate to the surface. It's a great guidance system.

And now, what is it you most want to see in your life? In this world? In your heart?

Tell yourself all about it. Have fun with it. Go into it in detail. You are a co-creator. You are a constituent of this planet. Your vote counts. Vote for what you want. And then get to work creating it.

My self talk:

- This is what I want:

- This is how I want to feel:
- This is how I want the world to be like:
- This is how I want to be:
- I can guide myself with my inner words towards creating my right life, and towards living fully as myself.

Being satisfied with my own efforts

For years, I have been meditating to the guided meditations of Dr Joe Dispenza. At the conclusion to one of them, he says, "and be satisfied with your efforts." When I first heard it, it hit me hard. Sometimes at the end of a meditation, I criticize myself because my mind drifted away at some points, or I felt I could have tried harder, or done better. Which is kind of funny, because that goes against the whole point of meditation.

It made me realize that I wasn't satisfied with my own efforts, generally. I often felt rushed, like I needed to hurry up so that I could do more. At the end of each day, I felt unsatisfied with what I'd done and who I was.

Let's look at the concept of satisfaction. Synonyms of satisfaction are contentment, pleasure, happiness, sense of well-being, pride, sense of achievement, delight, joy.

Having any kind of relationship with someone who cannot be satisfied is exhausting and draining. Nothing is ever good enough for them. You may feel anxious around that person. I know that I really don't enjoy spending time with someone who cannot be satisfied, whether that's a lover, friend, boss, or neighbour. It's discouraging.

And that includes my relationship with myself. I was discouraging myself and making myself feel anxious with my own self talk. That's a hard way to be inside, to be unsatisfied with one's own efforts.

I'm choosing to change that. Now, I've started telling myself that whatever I did that day, it's good enough, and I'm good enough. I'm satisfied. Instead of trying to cram in one more thing, I let myself have a little free time and space to just breathe and be. How radical! How relaxing to just be satisfied. I haven't been practicing this very long, but already I feel more happiness with myself, more calm, more wanting to be with me.

My self talk:

- I am satisfied with my own efforts.
- I am good enough.
- I did my best and it's good enough.
- You don't need to do more, or be more.
- Just be yourself, your full, glorious, and inimitable self.

The boundaries of healthy empathy and compassion

With what's happening in the world, we are being called to have more empathy towards each other. It is true that the world needs more empathy, but not from highly sensitive women.

The thing about HSWs is that we already feel so much empathy. We are wired to process way more information than regular folks, and that includes other people's feelings. In fact, research shows that we think about how others feel and what they need more than we think about ourselves.

Our sense of empathy is on overdrive. If empathy is a muscle, we're world champion bodybuilders. What we need, as HSWs, is the ability to balance our needs with those of others, and to learn how to practice more compassion.

What's the difference between empathy and compassion? I'm glad you asked because they are very different. Here is the difference between empathy and compassion as I see it.

Say that someone you know has fallen into a big, dark hole. In a state of compassion, you love them and you are of service to them if that's possible for you. You are present. You can throw down a ladder and encourage them to climb up. You can drop down a care package with food, a flashlight, blankets. You get what I'm saying. You remain solidly grounded in yourself and firmly within boundaries, while still loving them and acting compassionately.

In a state of hyper-empathy, we feel so bad for this person, we feel their suffering or pain. We think it's our job to fix it or save them. We jump down into the hole with them. Now there are two people stuck in this hole. That's not helpful to the other person, and not helpful to ourselves either. You are no longer in the center of your own life. You are living out someone else's life. If you have ever thrown yourself into someone else's hole, you know that it's really of no help ultimately. Plus, it's rather exhausting and confusing.

While I'm in this hole, while I'm in this other person's life, who's taking care of my life? Who's keeping it on course? Imagine a boat captain stuck down in the galleys while the vessel has no one holding the helm. There's no way to stay on course if you are not managing your own life.

Other people are way too much on a highly sensitive woman's radar. We can adjust our empathy dial and choose wisely when we help and how much we help. We can practice healthy empathy with boundaries and healthy compassion with boundaries too. We can be attuned to the needs of others, while ensuring that our own needs are front and center. It is from a grounded center that we can move into the world and be of service to others. Think of it like a wheel. You are the center. The spokes extend to where you put your love, attention, and energy. You, my beautiful, empathetic, highly sensitive woman, remain firmly in the center.

My self talk:

- I love myself and my life.
- I keep myself on my radar.
- I practice healthy empathy with boundaries, and healthy compassion with boundaries.
- I am just as important and as precious as other people.

- My life needs me to stay at the helm of it.
- There are so many ways that I can be compassionate, empathetic, and loving and still stay in the center of my own life.

Bring your attention to good news

If you keep up with the news now on offer 24/7, it does seem like it's a very scary time to be alive. Many people are scared and anxious. I don't need to remind you about all the alarmist news headlines because you are reading and hearing about them so much already.

Is what is presented in the news really reflective of what's happening? Surely, at minimum, it presents only one side of our big human story, a skewed view of the world as a scary place. I'm not saying that devastating things don't happen, but the world is also a place filled with wonderful people, events, comebacks, healings, turnarounds, transformations, and miracles. And it is certainly filled with many ordinary, peaceful days.

The problem is that good news rarely makes the news. It's just ignored. If one out of ten people has a problem, that's the person you will hear about. You won't be hearing about the nine people doing well.

I trained and worked as a journalist. There is a concept called "news hooks" – it means that journalists are looking for certain elements that they believe make a good story, a story that will be popular and sell ads. Fear, conflict, and violence are popular and powerful news hooks. People tune into the news way more when there is drama. Yes, there is an element of education in the news, but there is a much stronger element of wanting to attract the biggest numbers of people to sell ad revenue. And one way to attract people is to freak them out.

As highly sensitive women, we don't just shrug off the news like many less sensitive people can. Other people's suffering impacts us greatly. Archbishop Desmond Tutu reads the newspaper every day so he can know who is in need of prayers. That seems to be a great reason to follow the news. The other day, as I listened to the traffic report on the car radio, I wondered why we don't send love and well wishes to the people who have had accidents. It would be so healing if we sent love to everyone who is suffering instead of just mentioning the calamity they have suffered. We can do that in our hearts.

You get to decide what you focus on, where you bring your attention. With your self talk, you can remind yourself to notice the good, acknowledge it, and celebrate it. It's all around us! But it's not as attention-grabbing as drama, so you need to seek it out and give it a chance to make an impression on you.

Here is some good news to think about:

- Sea turtles are making a comeback from extinction. Humpback whales, too, going from a few hundred to 25,000.
- Billions of people are healthy and well today.
- Children who have healed are now playing outside with their friends.
- Dedicated groups and individuals are caring for their communities.
- People are enjoying the sun on their faces today.
- Teachers are giving their all to our children.
- Many people are in love – with their partners, with their pets, with life, with themselves.
- Young adults are graduating from university – it still remains an incredible achievement!

- 4,855 people waited in line in the rain for hours to take a stem cell test to help save a 5-year-old boy with a rare cancer.
- Firefighters extinguished fires and saved lives today.
- In pooch news, the Netherlands has become the first country with no stray dogs.
- Great news for our bees: London has created a green corridor of flowers; Holland planted green roofs on their bus stops as bee refuges; and a vaccine was developed in Finland to keep bees healthy and well.
- In one Indian village, they plant 111 trees each time a baby girl is born. So far, they have planted more than 350,000 trees.
- In personal good news, I saw five majestic bald eagles fly across the sky today. The sight filled me with awe and gratitude. Last week, my chiropractor made my neck feel so much better. Two weeks ago, my close friend happily married a kind, loving, strong, and generous man.

And if you want more good news, you have the power to do good and to care more and to love more, so that there will be more good news.

My self talk:

- I notice and celebrate the good inside of me, and all around me.
- There is amazing good news every day.
- I am contributing to the good.
- I am safe.
- I am grateful to be alive.

Earthing to soothe our nervous systems and calm down

Anxiety used to be like a pursuer I couldn't shake. Wherever I went, it was either by my side or not far behind. It was like travelling with the most uncomfortable travelling companion. Though I was high-functioning and looked Zen on the outside – most of the time – some days I was jittery and climbing out of my skin. Now, I feel a wonderful state of inner calm. And when I don't, I make it a priority to calm my system without delay.

Here's something that I do when I feel anxious, nervous, or overwhelmed. It's easy and everyone can do it. In the summer, I go lie right on the grass, preferably with my shoes off, and in the colder months, I find a big solid tree and I sit with my back against its trunk. I also will go to the beach and put my bare feet in the sand. Within 15 to 20 minutes, I will begin to sigh, big heaving sighs that are letting out tension. I know that it's kicking in. Then a calm will come over me. By the time I'm ready to get up, I'm a new person. I've been known to do this twice on a really tough day.

This practice is called earthing or grounding. By doing this, we connect to the electrical energy of the earth. They say there's a host of benefits to doing this, like improved blood pressure and lower stress levels, and I believe it. What I experience firsthand is the power this has to bring me back to me. When I'm in a calm and grounded state, I remember who I am. I can feel who I really am. In a way, when I'm anxious or overwhelmed, I am no longer myself. I can no longer feel love, or gratitude, or being present. I'm like a tiger in a cage looking for an exit.

Research has shown that it takes about 20 minutes for an over-aroused nervous system to calm itself and regain balance and coherence. When I combine meditation or breath work with grounding, I can get back into balance even quicker.

When anxiety kicks in, it doesn't benefit me to wait to bring myself relief. The quicker I can get to grounding when I'm in a state of stress, the quicker I'm back in business. Unless I'm dealing with an emergency, I will give myself permission to put everything aside and go find a tree and chill out with it. Not doing that would be like cutting myself while making dinner and not doing anything to stop the bleeding because I think I'm too busy to deal with it.

Go ahead. Find a big, fat, solid tree, or a slim one that sways in the breeze. Whatever calls to you. Sit at its base. Put your back against it. I like to pull my hat down over my eyes. Then just sit there with the tree. Or go lie in the grass or on the sand with your shoes off. This is earthing time. No cell phone. No reading. Be still. Give your nervous system a chance to relax, however many minutes that takes. Everything else can wait. You are connecting right now with the earth, with your self. This is a gift that we have as HSWs – we can feel this soothing energy and lean deeply into it.

My self talk:

- I give myself permission to take the time to calm my system.
- There are practices that help me feel inner peace.
- I can absolutely lower my anxiety levels.
- I can come back to myself and be free.

Asking the inner voice of anxiety to tone it down

A most important thing to keep in mind when it comes to self talk is that you have voices inside. We all do, whether we realize it or not. Some are more prominent than others, and some are hardly ever heard at all. And you, as the consciousness, are the one who listens. You are not one of the voices. You are the witness to it.

Think of yourself as the orchestra leader, and all your voices are the musicians. One's playing the violin, another is playing the cello, one's playing the piano, and one's on the triangle. (That's a sweet, kind one you need to be quiet to hear.)

Sure, you can let them all play willy-nilly, but you can also direct them to create more harmony and more beautiful music. You can orchestrate them. You can direct one to stop playing or to play much less loud.

That's exactly what I did the other day. I think there was a perfect storm of circumstances brewing that led to the moment when I started feeling anxious. I had been very busy. I had given loads to my family and community and hadn't spent enough time alone. I was tired. I had PMS symptoms on high during this period of perimenopause. I forgot all about a favour I had promised to do a friend, and I was filled with regret and worry about letting her down.

I was filled with anxious energy, and this time it was very tenacious, no matter what I tried. I was stuck in the feeling-thinking loop and was having trouble quieting my mind and my emotions.

Then I remembered that I am the orchestra conductor. It was obvious that I had a voice screaming out inside – a little like if my drum player was hitting the drum non-stop at full volume.

My inner voice of anxiety had been triggered by a stressor. It can be an event, an emotion or sensation in my body, or something I've told myself, or I can also be chemically or hormonally out of balance, like right before my period. Or I may have made lifestyle choices that had woken her up, like too much caffeine or sugar, too little sleep, or too much work.

I started by asking this voice to tone down. If she was agitated to an 8 or 9 out of 10, let's say, I asked her to tone it down to a 2 or 3. I said that she was making it very hard for me to think straight or to understand anything because the anxious energy going through my body was way too strong. The inner voice of anxiety responded by toning it down. I immediately felt somewhat calmer, and I sighed in relief. My shoulders dropped.

I thanked this voice for toning it down. I told it that I loved it. I also asked it what its message for me was, and I promised that I would take this message into consideration. Then I listened to anything that came to me. The message was that I was taking on too much once more, and that the voice wanted more free time to just be. There was lots of wisdom there underneath the screaming.

The last thing you want to do when you are feeling anxious is to abandon yourself. This little voice inside is scared and needs your presence, protection, care, and love. The inner voice is innocent and good. It is not its fault that it is nervous and fearful. There is part of you that can stand by yourself even as another part is distressed. Two parts of you can show up at the same time: the part that is anxious and the part that is powerful, steady, and caring. You are resourceful enough to be able to hold space for yourself that way.

My self talk:

- My inner voice of anxiety is triggered. I can ask it to tone it down.
- I can restore calm and quiet to my system.
- I can care for myself.

Declutter your self talk for freedom and inner peace

I recently had a bout of insomnia, waking up in the middle of the night for a few hours. I'm not sure why. It could have been from within, hormones, or old stories that are coming up. Or it could be from without – the energy of all that is happening in this world is affecting me. Or a combination of both. I don't know.

What I do know is that it triggered old stories. I dislike not being able to sleep with a passion. If I let myself go, I can make a way bigger story out of it than it really is. And I made up this a huge story. Poor me. Awake in the night, trolling the house like some forlorn ghost not getting her beauty sleep. I was quite ridiculous, if I may say so myself.

Because really, when I check myself and don't tell myself a story, it's quite peaceful in the night. Everyone is sleeping and quiet. I can read or meditate, and I've even gotten myself out of bed inspired to write. It's pretty sweet. And sure, the next day I am not in my best form, but it's generally ok.

My old inner story about not sleeping is irrelevant to what is really happening. It's completely exaggerated. It dates from other times in my life when I had trouble sleeping. These inner stories are out of date. They need to be decluttered so that I can replace them with stories that support me and my life. I've been on a roll to declutter both my home and my inner words. Just like I don't need to keep objects that I no longer use or love in my home, I don't need to keep inside me words and stories that no longer serve me.

Think of it like this. My old insomnia story is like an old CD with music that I no longer like or need. But this CD starts playing on its own whenever it decides. That's all it is. An old CD that starts playing on its own, and it plays and plays and plays the music, stuck in a loop, until I notice and turn it off.

This is what this voice says when I can't sleep:

This is terrible.

I won't be able to function well tomorrow with so little sleep.

Poor, poor me.

Why is this happening?

I don't feel good.

I'll get sick if I don't sleep enough.

And then, because this voice is agitated, it brings up all kinds of dire predictions and remembers dark moments of my life.

Esther Hicks calls that kind of self talk sloppy. That made me laugh. That's exactly what I'm inclined to do in the middle of the night when I can't sleep. My self talk is super sloppy. Meaning that I'm not taking care of it, I'm not managing it. I'm just letting it be whatever it wants to be. I'm just going along for the ride – which isn't very pleasant and is, frankly, a waste of my time and energy.

I know that no good comes out of sloppy self talk, so as soon as I notice, I switch to another voice because that's a power that I have. We all have that power. And I'll be honest here: When it comes to insomnia, this is not an easy task for me. I keep having to switch voices again and again and again. In a way, it's good practice, like doing your scales on the piano. It's also a good benchmark of the work and healing I still need to do around my self talk.

I remember that I'm not the voice who's distressed about not sleeping. I am the witness to it. I am the one listening to it. And I can choose to give myself love and compassion, and to stop listening to this broken old CD that's telling a story that's no longer true.

There's freedom in this, and inner peace.

I spoke to myself with another voice, a wiser, more grown-up voice, one that is way more mellow. This voice told me:

Everything is absolutely ok.

Let's talk about wonderful things in your life and what you are grateful for.

Maybe there's a good reason you are awake.

I'll give you a chance to rest tomorrow.

I love you.

So goodbye, old, irrelevant story. I'm decluttering you. I'm thanking you for your service, and letting you go so that I can replace you with a story about what a good sleeper I am, and how I always get the sleep that I need. And when I am awake, it's a positive story about how lucky I am to have this quiet space and time all to myself.

What old stories do you think you can do without? In my free self talk course, you can learn how to declutter old messages that no longer serve you and replace them with empowering and supportive self talk. Sign up here if you're ready to ditch old inner stories: https://selftalklove.lpages.co/self-talk-love-free-5-day-course/

My self talk:

- I can declutter my inner words, I can declutter my self talk.
- I don't need to carry around all the stories that have been following me for years.
- I decide what stories play in my head. I have that power.
- I am not the voice inside who is worried. I am the one who listens. And I can choose to listen to another voice and another story.
- I am not controlled by sloppy self talk.
- I give myself love and compassion no matter what story I'm telling myself.

A vacation from worry and multi-tasking

We had a little vacation one weekend in a hotel in our own city, 24 hours to wander around unscheduled and unhurried.

Before we left, I consciously told myself that I was leaving my to-do list and worries at home. I was giving myself a little break. I wanted to fully focus on enjoying the city with my family.

And it really worked. While I was there, I didn't think of my to-do list that never ends. I also didn't check email once and left my phone alone. I really gave all my energy to this little break. I came back feeling calm and centered. All it took was 24 hours.

I used to pride myself on my ability to multi-task. You should have seen us juggling away at our PR agency. I consider multi-tasking an old habit to break now. I think it harms me to dilute my focus like that. Studies show it actually is detrimental to my brain.

So instead of multi-tasking now, I try to do one thing after the other as needed. For sure, some days the heat is on, and it certainly is practical that I have that handy skill. As a rule, though, I live a different way now.

Just do one thing after the other as needed. If I give myself a chance to start my day off calmly and filled with as much serenity as possible, then the rest of the day stands a better chance of being like that, too.

My self talk:

- Just focus on what you are doing now.
- I do one thing at a time.
- It's ok to put down my load.
- It's ok to take a holiday from my worries and to-do-list.
- It's ok to just enjoy this moment.
- I give myself permission to just be right now.
- My worth is not attached to what I do. My worth is in who I am.

Being a witness to my feelings

I am often asked if self talk is affirmations. And certainly, affirmations are a component of self talk. Overall, self talk is the myriad of ways you communicate with yourself. Like a conversation, it's what you say and also how you listen.

Sometimes self talk is used to move away from something that is negative, to make it more bearable – like the way you may speak to yourself when you are feeling stressed and want to help yourself calm down.

Sometimes, it's to go towards something positive – like how you may encourage yourself to pursue a dream.

And sometimes, self talk is just to acknowledge what is going on, what your experience is. You are not trying to change it or fix it.

You become your own witness. In doing so, you connect with yourself. You are no longer alone, because you have shown up for yourself.

That happens when I tell myself what I am feeling. I show myself that I have noticed what is going on – just like you would with a good friend. Say you met your friend, and she felt sad. You would not ignore her. You may say something like this:

"I see how sad you feel. What is happening to you? Tell me about it."

When I do that for myself, it's like part of me relaxes because it has been noticed. We become one, as opposed to me ignoring part of myself.

Feelings are like messages that one part of you is communicating to another part. They are neither good nor bad. They are just messages hoping to be received and acknowledged. They are meant to come in and come out. We acknowledge them, we feel them, and they can be released. I can then raise my energy so that I can be in a state of higher feelings like joy, gratitude, and bliss.

I can tell you that the more time I spend in the company of elevated feelings like joy, gratitude, and bliss, the more my system calms down, and the more I feel at ease and at peace. My body gets flooded with feel-good hormones, and that makes me feel even better. It's like spending time in a spa. Spa time counterbalances the stresses of everyday life. Blissful feelings counterbalance the feelings of fear, sadness, overwhelm, and anxiety. And one day, the balance tips, so that you are feeling more joy, gratitude, and bliss in a day than anything else.

My self talk:

- I take time to touch base with how I'm feeling.
- My feelings transmit messages to me.
- I feel a wide range of feelings – that is a part of being human.
- I can elevate my energy and feel elevated feelings such as joy, gratitude, and bliss. The more I feel them, the easier they are to feel.

My guardian and friend, anger

When I got angry, I completely lost my cool. Think of the Hulk, and you get the picture.

My choices seemed to be to go with that huge energy and strike, or shove it down and let it dissipate. I didn't know what else to do. Basically, I struck out when I lost control, and I shoved it down when I was able to manage that.

Instead of anger helping me restore boundaries that had been crossed or protect myself or those around me, it would turn into a game of shame where I'd get angry, fling that anger out in a very aggressive way, then feel sorry afterwards. It's hard to feel dignified after a full-blown adult tantrum.

Sometimes, the Hulk did have its place – like when predatory men came too close. Nothing says "get out of my face" like the Hulk. But when dealing with friends and family that I love, not so much. So what to do?

The writings of Karla McLaren are helping me see anger in a new light. She writes: "Simply put, anger is a necessary and magnificent emotion that can improve your life and your relationships in astonishing ways." She calls anger the honourable sentry. It is there standing guard, protecting you and your boundaries, dignity, and honor.

I know that anger can be a wonderful informant and powerful catalyst. It helps me realize when my boundaries have been crossed and need enforcing. It protects me and those around me. Anger also helps me be more authentic. It propels me to speak up for myself and protect my rights. It can help me stand in a more empowered position. There is such a thing as healthy anger.

Knowing something in theory and knowing how to apply it to my life – the how-to – are two different animals. Think giraffe and platypus.

Just recently, I had a chance to practice, to put healthy anger into action, to go from thinking to doing. A friend crossed a line. I was upset and angry. Instead of slamming into him or swallowing it up, I calmly informed him that he had dishonored a boundary, and that I was angry. It came from a sense of dignity, and of love for me and for him. This gave us a chance to restore our relationship. I was able, as McLaren writes, to set my boundaries mercifully.

Anger and I are becoming friends now. I invited it over for tea. (Two sugars and a splash of milk for Anger, black for me.) I think my new friend is pretty cool.

When I think of anger as a gift, it opens up a whole new world of health: healthy emotions, healthy self-esteem, and healthy relationships. McLaren says the internal questions to ask yourself when anger arises are: "What must be protected? What must be restored?"

In my family, it was not cool to feel or display anger. I took that on. To not be ok with anger, to not be able to use your anger as a catalyst and energy, is like having an abundance of money but not having access to any of it.

We have a lot to be angry about – that's for sure. Violence, the destruction of our planet, sexual, physical, and emotional abuse, patriarchy, racism, starving children, homophobia – you get it, you live here too. The question is, what will we do with that anger? How will it serve us? Will we use it as a source of power and then rise above it to make the world a better, healthier, more loving and more balanced place? It's up to you and me.

My self talk:

- Anger is a healthy and much-needed emotion.
- I can use my anger in a skilful and intelligent way. It never needs to degrade others.
- I give myself permission to feel all my emotions.
- What needs to be protected? What needs to be restored?
- Anger is an amazing source of power.
- I enforce a boundary that you have crossed because I love us both.
- I can feel my anger and then rise above it.

You are good enough – in fact, you are perfect

"Ring the bell that still can ring, forget your perfect offering. There is a crack in everything. That's how the light gets in." This Leonard Cohen quote is another favorite of mine. I have cracks, for sure, but at the same time I am perfect. Let me explain.

We humans have a funny idea of perfection that's really hard to shake. Being perfect is not a clean bathroom floor, an A+ at school or at work, a flat tummy, a waxed bikini line, or a face without wrinkles. Perfection is not putting everyone's needs in front of your own, saying yes all the time, or forever chasing the upgrade to your life.

Perfection is what we are already. It is how we are born. We are all perfect, in a divinely human way. We are not fixer-uppers constantly in need of self help and amelioration. We are perfect already. What happens to us is that we get separated from this truth. We no longer know we are perfect. So it's not a question of getting fixed. It's a question of realizing who we are, of feeling it, of knowing it, of waking up to it. We are made of divine stuff, so how can it be otherwise? Perfection is love. The love that we are. The love that we feel. The love that we give others and ourselves.

You are perfect just the way you are as a highly sensitive woman. Your perfection cannot be compared to someone else's, for we are the same but also different. Your role, mission, vocation, calling, and gifts are different. Nobody else can play your role but you. The universe so wanted you to exist that it created you. As a good friend recently told me, your journey is equal to anyone's. You are needed, you belong, you are worthy, you are legitimate, you are perfect.

My self talk:
- I'm good enough.
- It's good enough.
- I am perfect.
- I am a perfect me. I was made to be me and that's the role I am playing in this lifetime. No one else can play it. If I don't do it, it goes unfilled.

The eagle's message of empowerment

As I walked in the forest behind my house, I suddenly heard a big rustling sound coming from a tree behind me. A huge bald eagle came majestically flying out of it. It was barely a few feet above my head. The eagle flew in a tight circle around me, a full 360 degrees, while looking me in the eyes. Then it soared away.

I stood there immobile for a long time, heart beating fast, transfixed. I had felt the eagle's enormous power. This was an extraordinary encounter. I knew the eagle had appeared for a reason, that it had a message for me.

I took the time to be quiet and to listen inside to what this message could be. What was the eagle telling me? What did I need to see, and understand?

Eagles can soar and see the big picture. Eagles are signs of having vision, of seeing what others cannot. What kept coming back to me was how powerful that eagle had felt, how strong.

I thought of my own inner power and how often I had diminished it, how often I had dimmed it. I have often played smaller than I really am. I have also doubted just how strong I am, how I am able to cope with disappointments, how I am able to carry on when things get tough.

When I sit quietly with myself, and I listen to my wise inner voice – the one which is underneath all the other voices chattering away – I can feel my own power, one that runs deep, one that is much bigger than just me. It is strong and very loving, too.

You have this power inside you. Take the time to feel it, to embody it. It is there for the taking. This power is there to support you on all your adventures.

One of your powers is your ability to choose your self talk. Kind, encouraging, and loving inner words empower you. When you criticize yourself, when you use inner words that are cruel and debasing, you lose energy, and some of your power with it. It's like a leak in a tire – you get deflated.

It's also in your power to learn new self talk skills and to choose to speak to yourself like a good friend would. Believe me, my sweet, if I could change my inner words, you can too. I was the queen of negative self talk. I was all kindness and "you can do it!" to others on the outside, but if you heard the thrashing that went on inside... ouch. I was giving away all the good powerful words to others.

When you are on your own side, when you stand by yourself with compassion and kindness even when you make mistakes or fail, your power increases because you are not divided against yourself. You are whole, and that is a very empowered way to be. Get a free worksheet for self talk power here: https://selftalklove.lpages.co/self-talk-love-speaking.../

My self talk:

- I take the time to listen to my inner voice.
- I am powerful.
- I am strong enough to do this.
- I trust in my inner power.

Tell yourself it is possible

Several years ago, I was in the gym with TVs blaring in the background when someone turned on the inauguration of President Obama. I hadn't thought much about the election until I saw him and his family in their gorgeous clothes – I still remember Michelle with that fabulous long yellow coat and olive-green leather gloves – outside in the cold. And suddenly it hit me, and it hit me hard. If Barack Obama could be elected, if it was possible for him, as an African American man, to become President of the United States, then it was possible that I would become a mother. I was hit with a surge of energy and hope. I believed it. I knew it was possible, deep inside me. I started moving on that elliptical machine with renewed vigour and a bounce in my step. Why not me indeed!

When I watched the inauguration, I was in the middle of a long fertility struggle, years of trying to become a mother. We'd been told the chances were slim, less than 5 percent. But what were the odds of Barack Obama becoming president? Surely, they had been slim like mine. And yet, there he was, looking proud, honoured, and strong. AHA! If it was possible for him, it was possible for me! It turns out that, in fact, it was possible for me!

What else is possible for me, for you, for us as a world?

It is certainly not the case that because something has been a certain way for a long time, it is meant to stay that way. It can change for the better. It is possible. Right now is a good time to tell yourself that it is possible. Whatever it is that you dream about, that you desire for your life, that you hold as your most sacred of intentions, it is possible.

May this be a time of opportunities, synchronicities, and possibilities for you.

My self talk:

- It is possible that love bloom.
- It is possible that our world be just and fair.
- It is possible to be peaceful.
- It is possible to be free.

- It is possible to reconcile.
- It is possible to heal.
- It is possible that my dream will come true.
- It is possible! It is possible! It is possible!

Numbing vs soothing

A few years ago, I went to give a workshop in a very remote retreat center. The road leading there was twisty turvy and I was nauseous for hours. There was no internet or cell reception and I worried about my daughter the whole time. Plus, I slept very poorly, haunted by nightmares that had me waking up punching and screaming.

After the retreat, I stayed for one night at a sweet little boutique hotel before making my way home. I sat in bed and turned on the TV, exhausted and overwhelmed. For hours, I watched ridiculous TV shows and ate a piece of cake. I had had enough. I was tuning out. Underneath it, though, I could still feel myself buzzing. Finally, I turned off the TV and picked up my journal. I started to just doodle in it, writing words that came to me. I decided to connect with myself instead of evading myself. It didn't take very long for me to feel much better, way calmer. The TV was numbing in a way, but it was also agitating.

What we feel, what we sense, and what we process as HSWs can be completely overwhelming to our systems. It may seem like too much, and many of us turn to drugs, alcohol, food, shopping, social media, binge-watching, or you name it. I sure did a lot of that. I just wanted to shut it all off, stop the input, pull the off switch for a while.

Then I discovered there's a big difference between soothing and numbing. When I numb myself, I want to divest myself of sensation. Think of anesthesia or being in the cold too long. To soothe is to relieve, to calm, and to comfort. They are quite different both in how I achieve each state and the benefits I receive from them.

When I am numb, I am lost to myself. As I take substances or sedate myself in other ways, I abandon myself. Part of me inside is in real need of help, and I'm kind of saying to it, "shut up. I don't want to hear what you have to say. I'm not interested in the fact that you are anxious and overwhelmed."

When I am soothed, I return to myself. I am present with myself. I hold my own hand until I can ease back into my real state. There's an immense benefit in its own right in just showing up for myself.

Often, it takes more effort to soothe than to numb. That's for sure. As I try to soothe a system that's like a rearing bronco, or that's frightened or overwhelmed, it's very uncomfortable. It can even seem unbearable. It takes about 20 minutes for an overwhelmed nervous system to calm down, so I have to be willing to be with myself until I can regain a state of calm. There are many ways that I can do this. I can take a warm bath, I can meditate, I can walk barefoot on the beach or in the grass, I can sit by a tree, I can listen to calm music, I can even dance. When I do this, I am putting calm, quiet, and gentleness in. The more I do it, the more skilful I will get at doing it and the quicker my nervous system will respond to it.

Soothing is way more powerful for me now than numbing. It enables me to feel good, relaxed, present, even if I'm tired.

If you have been numbing yourself or self-medicating, it's not your fault. There is no blame at all. Please don't beat yourself up about it. You have always done the best you can with what's available to you at that moment. There are a lot of tough energies in this world for HSWs to contend with and it takes time to become skilful at navigating them. You can learn to do it – that's for sure. Today is a new day. Right now is a new moment. You can choose to make a new decision, set a new intention for yourself and for your self-care.

My self talk:

- I take the time to soothe my system.
- I'm an HSW and I need specialized care.
- The advantages of being an HSW offset the challenges a million to one.
- If I do decide to numb myself, that's ok. Tomorrow is another day.

Knowing who I am

My daughter is a highly sensitive person, just like me. From this perspective, she knows exactly who she is. She is seen, and acknowledged, and validated.

When she was about five years old, she was invited to a birthday party in an art studio. They gave the kids brushes and had them whisk paint all over a large canvas on the floor. All the kids loved it except for my daughter, who started to cry. It was way too intense to be in a little room with all these kids laughing and screaming and throwing paint all over the place. I gently took her out of the room and brought her to a quiet corner where we could regroup. I knew exactly what was going on with her.

After that time, she became very selective as to which invitations she accepted. She knew that rowdy birthday games, or large gatherings, were not for her. She also knew at a young age that too much sugar doesn't suit her or that screen time after dinner will make her jittery at bedtime. She is also not suited to a packed, busy schedule or daily after-school activities. She needs loads of downtime and free play to recoup from school.

I am raising her to know who she is and what she needs. She is aware of herself. She can be proud to carry this trait. She's a gorgeous, highly sensitive girl, and I want her to know it.

In a documentary about highly sensitive people, Alanis Morrissette, one of us, said that her mother just didn't know how to deal with her and her sensitivity when she was a child. Many of us grew up like that. We were either raised by parents who weren't highly sensitive or by highly sensitive parents who were not yet aware of who they were.

I remember, as a child, watching a movie with my family, none of whom carry our trait. There was a very violent scene. I screamed and ran to my room. My family just kept watching, completely confused by my reaction and finding it kind of amusing.

My mother and I would get into arguments when she would drag me to a mall and I would make us leave way before she was ready. I just could not handle a moment more of that energy. Now, of course, I know why.

I would be far into adulthood by the time I discovered who I am. It was such a relief. I have seen this same relief in the faces of many women when they realized who they are.

It's amazing the difference it makes in life when we know ourselves. We can stand with so much more power. We can take action to create lives that suit an HSW. We can also stop comparing ourselves to others. An apple is an apple. An orange is an orange. And we are the sweetest, most extraordinary, and distinctive fruit there is.

My self talk:

- I know who I am.
- I am proud to be an HSW.
- I live my life in ways that suit me and my nature.

Permission to give myself what I need as an HSW

Here's what I need as an HSW to be well, to be rested, to be at ease, to be living my right life. I give myself permission to take care of myself in these ways.

I need time without plans so I can be free to engage in whatever calls me at that moment – and that may be doing sweet nothing.

I need time to connect with myself in the quiet and freedom of my heart.

I need to quiet my mind. Let it settle like a kite that gently lands on grass after whirling in heavy winds.

I need time to listen to what my inner voice of intuition is whispering. "Come close. I have something true and good to tell you," it says.

I need meaning in my work. I must follow its call. Only I can know what my calling and vocation are. As the Buddha said, "Your work is to discover your work and then, with all your heart, to give yourself to it."

I need nature, the ocean, trees and flowers, and the breeze in the wind chime.

I need to be reminded of the good people do, of acts of compassion and mercy. I want to know all about the intimate details of kindness. I want to revel in it. I turn towards this with all my power, like a plant reaches for the sunlight on the windowsill.

I need to go offline and disconnect from electronics. I am not wired (pun intended) to be at ease with too much of it.

I need relationships where I can connect on a deep heart and soul level, laugh and be at ease, and be myself.

I need gentleness, humour, and optimism in my media choices. I need to stay away from entertainment that is filled with words, images, and stories that are not in my highest good and don't celebrate life.

I need nutritious foods that nurture health, strength, and a sense of calm.

I need to be with people I love, and to be with people who emanate positive and loving energy.

I need loads of sleep. Blessed, restorative sleep. I protect my sleeping hours. They are not the first to get cut out on busy days. In fact, the busier I am, the more I need to sleep.

I need my home to be a "sanctuary from the loudness of the world" – thank you, Marianne Williamson, for these beautiful words.

I need to feast my eyes on the good, and true, and beautiful. Beauty will indeed save the world.

I need to move my body. It's my physical vessel and it loves to dance, stretch, swim, walk, and run.

I need to meditate and contemplate. As it's no big deal to brush my teeth every day so they remain strong and healthy, it's no big deal to get in touch with my inner self every day so I remain strong and healthy.

I need help at times. I need teachers, and healers, and therapists, and neighbours, and friends.

I need to be the object of my own affection, to treat myself like a friend, to show myself that I matter.

What do you need to nurture your highly sensitive nature?

A few words in closing (because I take such delight in us)

I hope that you now see what I see in you, in me, in us, in our clan of highly sensitives. When you sum it all up, the whole kit and caboodle, no other conclusion is possible than the realization that we are remarkable.

We've been gifted with this trait of high sensitivity. It's a gift that necessitates some rearrangements and arrangements for sure. A Maserati is trickier to drive than a Chevrolet, but no one is going to argue against the inherent value, power, and style of that rare and exquisite Italian sportscar. We sure are not Chevrolets – thank goodness for that.

If car analogies don't do it for you, think of an orchid, an exquisite flower that flourishes under care. With the knowing you now have, you can become the gardener of your own body, mind, and spirit, ensuring that you keep giving yourself what is needed to bloom as a treasured orchid. What could be more worthwhile in this life than falling in love with yourself? When self-love is the way you move and groove, when it's your way of being, you become an example of pure grace and it serves all humankind.

Research shows that the brains of sensitives are extremely neuroplastic. We are masters of growth and change. We learn really fast and adapt easily. If you haven't been tending to your garden until now, no worries, no guilt. Start right now – any way that calls to you.

As you move on with this awareness and love for whom you are, you will cultivate discernment and know what is just right for you as a sensitive. Think of yourself as a matchmaker, like the ones of old in the shtetls. Life success rested in the compatibility of the match. You have the wisdom to match yourself with the right persons, places, situations, and work.

With great compassion, put down the burdens that aren't yours to carry. Shine that HSW light and power onto yourself first, and as you do so, it will light the way for others.

If you'd like to take a deeper dive with me into the transformational power of positive self talk, contact me at maryse@selftalklove.com and I will sign you up for my free online five-day course.

Be well, dear HSW, and thanks for reading.

Thankfulness

How grateful I am for all the help that I received writing this book, and on my path to recognizing my high sensitivity and embodying it with joy.

Lori-Ann Speed, you were the first to tell me about who I really was and to point me to several great resources, including Dr Elaine Aron's work.

Therapist Pamela Catapia taught a series of Saturday classes on high sensitivity. It was the first time I found myself in a room knowing that I was surrounded exclusively by highly sensitive individuals. We totally got each other. Pamela provided so much wisdom, insight, and great tools.

I am made this way by Divine design and for this I am so grateful.

My husband Robert provides a solid and calm rock onto which I can grow and be my best highly sensitive self in joy, safety, and freedom.

Eloise is my teacher. How can I not embrace my own high sensitivity as I celebrate yours?

You wouldn't be Eloise if you weren't highly sensitive, and that just wouldn't do.

A shout out to all the highly sensitive men who are awakening and realizing that this trait is a superpower and that they are so needed in the creation of a new world. I have met several of these exemplary men. Thank goodness you exist.

Thank you Sara for the strong copy editing skills that you bring to my work.

Avital, you have once again designed a beautiful cover for my book. I love your work and I am grateful to call you my friend.

Resources

HSP-focused psychology

Pamela Catapia is a therapist who specializes in working with highly sensitive individuals.

Dr Elaine Aron provides the science and information about our high sensitivity. Her website also includes self-tests and a wonderful collection of books, including The Highly Sensitive Child, which I found very helpful and validating.

Blog

Highly Sensitive Refuge

This is a great blog written by some of us. Loads of tips and recognition.

Books

The Highly Sensitive Survival Guide

This book is filled with practical tips on how to remain calm, sane, and safe, such as what to pack when travelling.

Dodging Energy Vampires: An Empath's Guide to Evading Relationships That Drain You and Restoring Your Health and Power

This book by Dr Christiane Northrup provides guidance on how to care for and protect yourself as an HSW.

Speaking to Yourself with Love: Transform Your Self Talk Workbook

Go from self-critical to self-kindness with this beauty of a workbook written by Maryse Cardin. It is filled with beautiful illustrations and space to write, draw and doodle.

About the author

Maryse Cardin is an author, workshop leader, speaker, communication university teacher, and very proud HSW. Her passion and work focus on positive self talk, self-esteem, and unconditional love. Right on! Visit her at www.selftalklove.com and www.facebook.com/selftalklove

Made in United States
North Haven, CT
05 October 2021

10160027R00095